ANTICORRUPTION IN THE HEALTH SECTOR

ANTICORRUPTION IN THE HEALTH SECTOR

STRATEGIES FOR TRANSPARENCY AND ACCOUNTABILITY

Edited by

Taryn Vian, William D. Savedoff
and Harald Mathisen

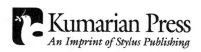

Kumarian Press
An Imprint of Stylus Publishing

Anticorruption in the Health Sector: Strategies for Transparency and Accountability

Published in 2010 in the United States of America by Kumarian Press, 22883 Quicksilver Drive, Sterling, VA 20166, USA

The text of this book is set in 10/12.5 New Baskerville

Editing and book design by Aptara

The paper used in this publication meets the minimum requirements of the American National Standard for Information Sciences—Permanence of Paper for printed Library Materials, ANSI Z39.48-1984

Library of Congress Cataloging-in-Publication Data

Anticorruption in the health sector : strategies for transparency and accountability / edited by Taryn Vian, William D. Savedoff, and Harald Mathisen.
     p. ; cm.
  Includes bibliographical references and index.
  ISBN 978-1-56549-338-4 (cloth : alk. paper) – ISBN 978-1-56549-337-7 (pbk. : alk. paper)
  1. Medicine–Corrupt practices.   2. Hospitals–Corrupt practices.
3. Medicare fraud.   I. Vian, Taryn.   II. Savedoff, William D.
III. Mathisen, Harald.
   [DNLM: 1. Fraud–prevention & control.   2. Health Care Sector.
3. Health Care Reform.   W 74.1 A629 2010]
   RA410.5.A63 2010
   364.16′3–dc22

                                               2009048966

Contents

Illustrations

Preface: A Guide to Effective Anticorruption Reform

Struggling against corruption can be a thankless task. Despite the efforts of resourceful people around the world to help their countries overcome corruption, headline-grabbing scandals never seem to end. Occasionally, those who rise to challenge corruption are recognized as heroes, but all too frequently, they are harassed, lose their jobs, or even end up fearing for their lives.

Although this predicament can be discouraging, this book challenges the pessimism that too often clouds anticorruption reform efforts, holding that more effective interventions are within reach, particularly those that work strategically in particular institutions or sectors. By describing anticorruption strategies for the health sector that have proven successful, we demonstrate that it is possible to combat corruption effectively.

The stakes could not be higher. Corruption in the health sector is literally a matter of life and death for poor people in developing countries who experience the consequences of fraud and abuse: long trips to reach critical health-care services, missing drugs, or the high cost of paying bribes. Combating corruption in the health sector also holds enormous promise in terms of building trust in public institutions and, therefore, building support to promote integrity in other sectors. Finally, the sums of money involved are so large, representing significant shares of national income, government revenues, and donor aid, that corruption cannot be ignored.

Fortunately, an emerging body of knowledge is helping to translate the findings of anticorruption research into operational anticorruption programs. Although we still have much to learn, a number of general lessons from this field are already proving useful for designing and implementing anticorruption reforms.

Avoid Blueprints, Please

Where do we begin? An intervention needs to be designed around a specific problem and context. Its effectiveness will always depend as much on a country's culture, history, institutional constraints, and capacities as it does on incisive analysis of the forms of corruption. Practitioners can either adapt relevant approaches from other places or recognize that they need to invent new ones.

Attempts to apply standardized "solutions" are far too common; following a blueprint without concern for the characteristics of a particular corruption problem in its own context is counterproductive. Learning from experiences in different countries and different sectors does not mean blindly replicating those experiences. Quite the contrary. Cultural norms, social institutions, and political processes all color how people view corruption and whether they are even willing to confront it, and local officials or activists can create unique solutions that take into account these local factors. Instead of looking at a corruption issue as a dichotomous, winner-take-all conflict between tradition and modernity, they can pay careful attention to local knowledge, eliciting local values that are compatible with improved integrity and better governance. Local actors should therefore assume the lead roles, tailoring their own approach to corruption. When domestic engagement and learning from abroad combine this way, the resulting reform process has a better chance of success.

Be Strategic and Target Interventions Wisely

What should we do? It is tempting to design comprehensive approaches that address every aspect of corruption. These may succeed in some instances, with appropriate and sufficient political will. However, the effort to do everything at once, whether at the national level or at the sector level, can also be counterproductive. Such broad strategies can lose momentum and end up with little impact; strategic and targeted approaches are likely to work better.

Targeted approaches can address defined problems in a particular sector with specific measures of progress and a manageable number of stakeholders. If actions are targeted within a broader sector strategy, they can also avoid becoming isolated or overly narrow. For example, introducing links between performance measures and budget expenditures can uncover public financial mismanagement and generate support for broader action; or tackling embezzlement of user fees in local facilities can be a first step, followed by actions to reduce theft of medications or bribes.

Make Anticorruption Reforms Part of the Mainstream

How should we proceed? Corruption is often a symptom of poorly managed public systems, so it makes sense to address it as part of mainstream reforms. If officials attend to corruption vulnerabilities whenever they make changes in public programs, anticorruption reforms can be advanced as part of the overall efforts to improve public policy. However, as with all attempts to "mainstream" cross-cutting issues (such as gender and human rights), it is important to respect the specialized knowledge of sector experts and clearly demonstrate that dealing with opportunities for corruption is integral to achieving the better sector performance to which they are dedicated.

Even in countries where people are highly mistrustful of state institutions, mainstreaming anticorruption efforts in a sector such as health care can also create positive momentum by identifying problems that are amenable to concrete and visible solutions. Whether initiating campaigns against counterfeit drugs in Nigeria or against informal payments in Albanian hospitals, committed individuals have shown that tackling corruption as part of a program to improve public management can be successful.

Exploit Opportunities

When should we start? The simplest answer is: now. In almost any circumstance, actions can be taken—large or small—to reduce the scope of corruption. But reformers should look in particular for social and political influences on the climate for reform and search for promising moments following an election, for example, or a high-profile scandal, an economic crisis, or a new senior-level appointment. International situations, such as a country's commitment to regional treaties or preparations for accession to an international alliance, can also be used as leverage to promote positive change.

Lack of political will is often cited as a reason why anticorruption efforts fail, and it certainly limits the available strategies. In such cases, rather than fighting corruption openly and relying on high-level leadership, indirect tactics may be preferable. For example, a program informing citizens about their legal rights to public health services might never mention corruption. However, as it aims to increase transparency, the program might bring to light cases of corruption that, once in the public eye, cry out for remedies and generate public support for subsequent action. Thus, in some cases, programs may be more successful if they are not explicitly labeled anticorruption efforts.

Another tactic in the face of opposition is to mobilize new allies. Sometimes this means letting the public know how corruption compromises their access to health care or endangers lives. In other cases, it involves publishing details about public expenditures and whether they reach their intended beneficiaries. Professional associations can sometimes be persuaded to enforce standards of integrity, either through incentives and rewards or through public shaming. In countries that have signed and ratified international agreements, the courts or the press can be enlisted to hold legislative and executive branches of government accountable.

Introducing a Strategic Sector Approach

The lessons from anticorruption reforms show that we can make great strides by promoting integrity in specific sectors and institutions. The health sector is a key candidate for action because it has such direct impact on the well-being of citizens. The health sector may also have a better chance of success than other sectors because it can draw on a strong ethical tradition. If successful, anticorruption efforts in the health sector can then inspire efforts against corruption in other parts of society as well.

In this book, we do not intend to create more blueprints. Rather, we show that reform is indeed possible, and that the best way to achieve it is to approach the process with sensitivity to local cultures and practices while being well informed about what has worked in other places. We have therefore highlighted successful interventions wherever we found them. We hope that these stories, experiences, and lessons will inspire you and others to confront this critical challenge with optimism, confidence, and persistence.

Acknowledgments

The research and analysis undertaken by contributors to this book received special support and encouragement from the U4 Anticorruption Resource Centre at the Chr. Michelsen Institute in Bergen, Norway. U4's mission is to assist donor practitioners in more effectively addressing corruption challenges through development support, working closely with eight development agencies: Norad (Norway), DFID (United Kingdom), CIDA (Canada), GTZ (Germany), MinBuZa (the Netherlands), Sida (Sweden), BTC (Belgium), and AusAID (Australia). Several of the chapters in this book first appeared in a slightly different format as case briefs on the U4 website (www.u4.no).

BTC, the Belgian agency for development cooperation, has graciously provided a grant that made it possible to add knowledge and update earlier research for this book. In addition, the International Health Department of the Boston University School of Public Health, a school committed to furthering innovation in the practice of public health, has been a steady supporter of our work and the notion that corruption is a public health problem that must be addressed by public health professionals.

We are very grateful, as well, to several individuals who assisted us in the preparation of the book. Rich Feeley and Lucy Honig provided excellent and insightful comments on early drafts of key chapters. Amanda Makulec skillfully handled myriad details in helping to prepare the final manuscript. Special thanks go to Kirsty Cunningham at U4 for providing exceptional copyediting of chapters. And finally, we are grateful for the encouragement and valuable advice of Jim Lance, editor and associate publisher at Kumarian Press, who guided us through the publishing process.

PART ONE

Taking Funds From
Public Coffers

CHAPTER 1

Introduction: Closing Opportunities for Corruption in the Health Sector

Taryn Vian, William D. Savedoff and Harald Mathisen

In an Indian maternity ward, a nurse tells a mother that she has to pay a fee to see her newborn girl. She says the charge would have been higher if it had been a boy.

In Costa Rica, a member of Congress is offered thousands of dollars if he will introduce legislation to approve a Finnish loan for the social security institute to import hospital equipment.

In Cameroon, a local committee applies for a grant to build a health post. With the committee's consent, the village leader increases the grant request to include materials to improve his own house.

In Albania, a private doctor prescribes a medication that a patient does not need because he has made an arrangement with the next-door pharmacist to get a share of the price.

These real stories of health sector corruption show how people can abuse their power. When officials divert funds or take bribes, they violate a public trust. But many times, stories of corruption are not straightforward. Most people who engage in corruption—or activities that look corrupt—have ways of rationalizing their behavior with explanations that may appear legitimate. To the extent that others in society share those rationalizations, the definition of corruption becomes blurred. Was the nurse's income so low that she was justified in "taxing" the mothers for more pay? Was it appropriate to reward the village leader for his role in getting the health post by asking for more funds from the government, even if the added amounts were not disclosed?

We believe that the challenge faced by anyone concerned with public health policy is to address health sector corruption not only as an economic or political problem but also as a practice rooted in the everyday logic of social behavior. Whether we approach the question as public health specialists, health policy advisors, applied economists, government officials, politicians, or NGO managers, we cannot ignore corruption's role in health system failures and in poor health outcomes that persist despite increasing aid. This book provides a resource for those who design public health policies or implement health programs and who recognize that corruption is a threat to public health goals.

The Problem

Corruption is a serious problem for both rich and poor countries, threatening international development and eroding confidence in government. In the health sector, corruption is literally a matter of life and death, if hospitals crumble because of embezzled construction funds, if doctors extort under-the-table payments from patients who cannot afford to pay, and if corrupt regulators allow fake drugs to flood markets. Although corruption can be found in every country, citizens in lower-income countries are more likely to experience corruption when they interact with public officials, and there is growing evidence that the effects of corruption on the health and welfare of citizens may be more harmful in poorer countries. These factors make corruption an important global health issue.

Defined as "abuse of public or entrusted power for private gain," corruption in the public sector occurs when a government agent who has been given authority to carry out public service goals instead uses his or her position to further personal interests. The list in Table 1.1 contains some of the most common types.

Difficulties in defining and measuring corruption abound. For example, it is not always easy to agree on what is "abuse" of power. When underpaid clinicians accept informal payments given willingly by patients who can afford them, is this truly an abuse of power, or merely a coping mechanism to gain a living wage? It is also very difficult to measure corruption, since the practice is usually hidden.

Corruption as a Health Problem

Corruption becomes a health problem by reducing the amount of funds available to invest in health. Private companies—both domestic and foreign—are reluctant to invest in countries with high levels of corruption, which lowers overall economic growth. Stagnant economies have fewer funds available for government in general and less revenue available

Table 1.1 Selected list of corrupt practices and their impact

TYPE OF CORRUPTION	EXPLANATION	IMPACT
Informal payments	Payments given to health providers which are greater than "official" fees, or for services that are supposed to be free	Reduce access to care; undermine equity in access; increase financial burden on patients
Selling government posts	When a senior official requires a payment from government agents to secure or keep their position	Increases likelihood of unqualified staff; people may feel pressure to abuse power in order to finance the "purchase" of their job
Absenteeism	Stealing time by not coming to work, or private practice during work hours	Reduces access to and provision of services
Bribes	Money or something of value promised or given in exchange for an official action	Bribes in medicines registration, selection, and procurement can result in high cost, inappropriate, or duplicative drugs, or subtherapeutic or fake drugs allowed on market
Procurement corruption	Encompasses many types of abuse including bribes, kickbacks, fraudulent invoicing, collusion among suppliers, failure to audit performance on contracts, etc.	Procurement corruption raises the price paid for goods or services, thus increasing inefficiency; goods and services may not even be needed, may not be delivered, or may be of substandard quality
Theft or misuse of property	Stealing or unlawful use of property such as medicines, equipment, or vehicles, for personal use, use in a private medical practice or resale	Results in higher unit costs; stock-outs of drugs, interruptions in treatment, or incomplete treatment; antibiotic resistance. Can impede access to care as patients stop coming to facilities

(Continued)

Table 1.1 (*Continued*)

TYPE OF CORRUPTION	EXPLANATION	IMPACT
Fraud	Deliberate misrepresentation with intent to secure unlawful gain. False invoicing; "ghost" patients or services (billing for patients who do not actually exist, or services not actually rendered); diversion of accounts receivables into a private account, etc.	The siphoning off of resources may result in insolvency of insurance funds; lower quality of care; denial of care for some patients or failure of programs to achieve results
Embezzlement of user fee revenue	Stealing or using funds that belong to an employer or a government agency	Less funding available for services; lower quality of care

to the health sector. Even within the health sector, decisions on allocating funds may be distorted by people who want to enrich themselves because it is easier to solicit a large kickback on a hospital construction contract or on the purchase of expensive, sophisticated medical equipment than on primary health-care programs such as immunization and family planning.

Corruption in the health sector also has a direct negative effect on access and quality of patient care. As resources are drained from health budgets through embezzlement and procurement fraud, less money is available to pay salaries and fund operations and maintenance. This can demoralize staff, lower the quality of care, and reduce the availability and utilization of services. Studies have shown that corruption has a negative effect on health indicators such as infant and child mortality (Gupta et al. 2002) and there is evidence that reducing corruption can improve health outcomes by increasing the effectiveness of public expenditures (Azfar 2005).

A review of research on informal payments found evidence that informal payments for care reduce access to services by making care less affordable, especially for the poor (Lewis 2007). In Azerbaijan, one study estimated that about 35% of births in rural areas take place at home, mostly because of high charges for care in facilities where care was supposed to be free (World Bank 2005), while in Armenia, families are forced to sell livestock or assets, or borrow money from extended family and community members, in order to make the necessary informal payments to receive care (Emerging Markets Group 2005).

Bribes to avoid government regulation of medicines have serious negative effects on health. Allowing medicines of subtherapeutic value to be sold can contribute to the development of drug-resistant organisms and increase the threat of untreatable pandemics. Corruption in the form of theft or diversion to private pharmacies can lead to shortages of drugs in government facilities, which may discourage people from seeking medical care. Procurement corruption can lead to inferior public infrastructure as well as high prices that government pays for materials, leaving less money for service provision.

A Framework for Assessing Vulnerabilities

Before intervening to control or prevent corruption, public health professionals—and anyone who wants to design, fund, or support interventions—need to understand why corruption happens in the health sector. What factors help explain the current pattern of abuses of public power or position for private gain in the health sector? How can we use this information to prevent and mitigate the serious and harmful effects of corruption?

One way of understanding corruption is to treat it as a rational choice. Individuals have legitimate personal interests but when they pursue those interests to the detriment of their social commitments and public responsibilities, it can result in corrupt behavior. People generally cross the line between honest and corrupt behavior when they have an opportunity to abuse their power at the same time that they feel pressured. They then devise rationalizations to justify their behavior (see Figure 1.1). Where individual rewards of corruption are great, and the likelihood of being caught and punished is low, people are more likely to engage in corruption. Some of the most fruitful corruption prevention strategies directly address this balance by making honesty more rewarding and corruption more costly. These strategies include raising salaries, developing performance-based rewards, strengthening professionalism and codes of ethics, increasing transparency, and raising penalties for corruption.

By understanding corruption in this way, we can identify aspects of the health system that can be changed to make corruption less likely. For example, any intervention to control pharmaceutical procurement corruption will have to address why there are opportunities, pressures, and rationalizations for abuse. However, the intervention that is appropriate to a particular context will depend on the level to which procurement is

Figure 1.1 Framework of corruption in the health sector

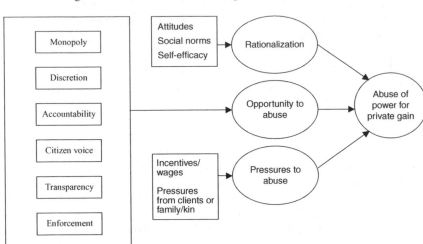

Health-care system and structure
- Insurance
- Payer–provider split
- Role of private sector, etc.

Type of abuse
- Financial fraud
- Procurement
- Informal payments, etc.

Resources
- High or low income
- Donor dependence, influx of funding

Source: Vian, T. 2008. Review of corruption in the health sector: Theory, methods, and interventions. *Health Policy and Planning* 23, no. 2:83–94.

centralized, the degree of professionalism and supervision for procurement officers, the quality and speed of the courts, and the culture of public service.

Studies have identified a number of ways that opportunities for abusing power can arise, along with measures to address them (Vian 2008). For example, if people are forced to pay bribes in order to get health-care services, the opportunity for abuse may occur because people have few alternatives (the health facility has a monopoly), the facility has no supervision (is unaccountable), or health-care workers believe that charging is acceptable (social norms). In each of these situations—monopoly, lack of accountability, and weak social service values—appropriate measures can be designed. Some of these factors and their application in fighting corruption are described in Table 1.2.

Summary of the Chapters

Fighting corruption requires strategies like these, which are grounded in theory, informed by evidence, guided by experience, and adapted to

Table 1.2 Factors and interventions

FACTOR	DEFINITION	POSSIBLE INTERVENTIONS
Institutional or system level		
Monopoly	A situation where there is only one provider of a service	Expand service delivery options so that citizens can choose facilities and services free of corruption; break up clan-controlled corruption
Discretion	Decision-making autonomy vested in a particular government agent	Clearly define roles and responsibilities of government agents and maintain appropriate controls on discretion to lessen opportunities for corruption
Accountability	Obligation or willingness to demonstrate effectiveness in carrying out goals and achieving results	Measure goals and results of government programs and share this information with internal and external monitors; require government agents to justify the level of performance achieved; punish nonperformance or corrupt behavior
Citizen voice	Channels and means for citizens to participate in government	Increase opportunities for citizens to choose priorities, review budgets, evaluate government performance, and lodge complaints
Transparency	Active public disclosure of information on roles, policies, process, objectives, and results of institutions	Disclose and disseminate information in ways that improve public deliberation, reinforce accountability of officials, stimulate citizen choice, and improve quality and fairness of public services

(Continued)

Table 1.2 (*Continued*)

FACTOR	DEFINITION	POSSIBLE INTERVENTIONS
Detection and enforcement	Steps used to detect corruption and to punish those caught	Increase investigation, policing, and surveillance; encourage investigative journalism; design and enforce legal/regulatory sanctions; develop professional codes of conduct and citizen watchdog organizations; support hotlines and whistle-blowing protections
Incentives	Compensation and other benefits that reduce pressure for engaging in corruption as a "coping mechanism"	Design health reforms to increase net pay and benefits for public employees; create strategies to reward good performance; improve working conditions so work is challenging and rewarding

Individual level (perspective of officials and citizens)

FACTOR	DEFINITION	POSSIBLE INTERVENTIONS
Attitudes	Overall evaluation of the behavior by officials and citizens (perceived pros and cons to participating in corruption)	Specify negative consequences of corruption; correct misinformation about the frequency of corrupt behaviors and address rationalizations; create awareness about role of government, citizen rights, and entitlements
Social and ethical norms	Value placed on public service; understanding of public or professional role; family/social expectations	Develop programs for public management education; create standards for integrity; support role models for ethical behavior
Self-efficacy	Confidence in one's ability to take action; temptation or personal pressures to engage in corruption	Demonstrate and model desired behavior; develop civic education to increase citizens' skills in explaining their problems and accessing government; increase knowledge of options for accessing services without bribes

context. Development agencies are promoting "mainstreaming" of anti-corruption, that is, incorporating anticorruption approaches in all sectors and at all intervention levels in order to achieve sustainable development results. But how do we adapt anticorruption principles to the particular context of health systems? What are the weaknesses in health systems that create vulnerabilities to corruption, and how can institutions be strengthened to reduce the likelihood of abuse?

The chapters that follow bring together theory and practice in mainstreaming anticorruption in the health sector. Each of the 12 essays discusses the consequences of specific types of corruption and presents real-world experience with anticorruption approaches tailored specifically to health sector vulnerabilities. The purpose is to help practitioners to gain practical insight into designing anticorruption strategies by learning how others have attempted to diagnose and address corruption challenges. The book is divided into four parts: Taking funds from public coffers; Demanding payment where services should be free; Manipulating procurement and drug supply; and Restoring integrity through transparency and accountability.

Taking Funds From Public Coffers

Hospitals account for more than 50% of health-care spending in many countries and are particularly susceptible to financial fraud. Chapter 2, "Fighting Fraud in Hospitals," describes three common types of fraud experienced in public hospitals in the developing world, including diversion of patient fee revenue, diversion of accounts receivable, and collusion between government procurement agents and suppliers. The chapter gives examples of how to prevent and detect fraud by strengthening internal control systems. Improved procedures may require additional investments, though the case is made that additional investment in fraud prevention and control is cost-effective.

One particular type of financial fraud, employee embezzlement of funds, may be a problem not only for hospitals but also for a range of government- and donor-funded programs. Chapter 3 tells the story of how embezzlement occurred in a donor-funded research program in Africa, exploring the systemic weaknesses that created opportunities for corruption as well as the pressures on individuals and their rationalizations. The chapter discusses how a donor should react when corruption is detected, and how actions depend on local environment and context. The authors observe that most donor projects have experienced similar losses and recommend enhancing intra-organizational learning.

Chapter 4 explores in depth the problem of theft of user fee revenue. Many countries in the developing world still rely on user fees to help fund health services. Although official user fee revenue often represents less than 5–10% of health-care spending, these funds may help to pay for continuous supply of medicines in decentralized facilities or to motivate staff through approved bonus payments. Automated information systems have proved helpful in reducing the loss of user fee revenue from unauthorized exemptions or diversion by cashiers. The chapter describes the experience of a Kenyan hospital that introduced policy and system changes to reduce theft of user fees. The author explains the incremental process that hospital managers used to continually improve systems and introduce responsible stewardship. The success of the program is linked to factors such as strong leadership commitment and the willingness and ability to discipline staff.

Demanding Payment Where Services Should Be Free

The two chapters in this part provide insights to the extent and causes of the problem of informal payments and possible policy solutions. While many studies have documented patient views on informal payments, few studies have explored the views of the practitioners who accept the payments. Chapter 5 explores this important and little-studied perspective by reviewing a qualitative study of informal payments conducted among health workers in Tanzania. The authors describe the nature of the informal payments and their potential impacts on access to and quality of health-care services. They also analyze policy implications of anticorruption strategies such as the need to compensate for the loss of informal revenue, ways to disseminate information to the public to increase support for reforms, and punishments for having extorted informal payments.

Chapter 6 continues the discussion of policy reforms, reviewing experiences in four countries that have tried to reduce informal payments: Albania, Kyrgyz Republic, Cambodia, and Armenia. The authors discuss the pros and cons of formalizing fees as well as alternative methods of deterring informal payments *without* charging fees.

Manipulating Procurement and Drug Supply

The third part of the book explores the important problem of corruption in procurement and drug supply. Pharmaceuticals alone can represent 30% or more of health-care spending. Along with other medical supplies, they are vulnerable to abuse through procurement fraud and theft.

A common explanation for corruption is that personnel are not well paid. Chapter 7 explores evidence from Latin American hospitals on low pay as a factor causing corruption in procurement. The author finds that while low pay of procurement agents is associated with corruption, higher paid workers may also be corrupt. Strategies to prevent corruption in pharmaceuticals procurement must therefore incorporate other factors in order to be effective, such as increasing the probability of getting caught and the magnitude of penalties. Implications for monitoring systems are also discussed.

Chapter 8 provides a detailed analysis of corruption in pharmaceutical distribution systems—the supply chain for storing and distributing drugs from warehouses to service delivery points. The author looks at both the theft of drugs and the diversion of supplies meant for the public market into private channels. The chapter explains how the US President's Emergency Plan for AIDS Relief (PEPFAR) and related projects are working to secure the supply of HIV/AIDS drugs from theft and counterfeiting. It also discusses specific interventions undertaken by a private drug distributor in South Africa to prevent corruption, resulting in loss rates well below the average for developing countries.

Chapter 9 discusses transparency and the impact of information on hospital procurement corruption in Argentina and Bolivia. It describes how active supervision by local health boards constrained corruption in Bolivia. It also tells what happened in Argentina when the government tried to limit opportunities for corruption in supply procurement by publishing the prices paid by different hospitals. After analyzing the results, the author cautions that transparency alone may not be a sustainable anti-corruption strategy. Unless there are consequences attached to identified malpractice, monitoring and publicizing information will not guarantee sustained improvements.

The link between transparency and accountability is also the subject of Chapter 10, which identifies ways in which information technology can improve transparency and increase accountability in procuring HIV/AIDS medicines. The chapter describes how international partners concerned about waste and corruption in pharmaceutical procurement have supported the development of a price monitoring system using public data. The authors present two transparency tools: price outlier analysis and country benchmarking, which can be used to spark public debate and pressure for action.

Restoring Integrity Through Transparency and Accountability

Fighting corruption is a complex undertaking, but there are steps policymakers and citizens can take to prevent corruption. This final part reviews several approaches to increasing transparency and accountability, looking in particular at financial indicators, special studies of public expenditures, and budget transparency.

Chapter 11 analyzes the role of transparency in promoting accountability and stakeholder engagement in the health sector. The author argues that health professionals need to develop transparency goals and tools adapted to their own context and the culture in which they are working, and to determine the best ways of communicating information to achieve transparency in different organizational settings. The chapter reviews concepts of information disclosure, right to know, and means of disclosure, highlighting the need to go beyond "generalities" and get very specific about who is owed what kind of information for what purpose. The chapter provides examples of how transparency can be achieved in budgets, procurement and delivery of medicines, human resources management, and quality of patient care.

Presenting the experience of district health management teams in South Africa, the authors of Chapter 12 assess the advantages and challenges of integrating utilization data and financial data to measure accountability in the use of funds. This type of integration of performance data with financial information is at the heart of performance-based budgeting systems being promoted worldwide as part of public finance reform. Chapter 12 describes the types of questions that were raised by the data, and how they shed light on operational issues and potential vulnerabilities to corruption.

Finally, Chapter 13 describes how budget transparency can help to ensure that public funds are used appropriately, thereby limiting the scope for corruption. The chapter examines ways to establish citizens' rights to information, to make the information easier to use, and to establish accountability to citizens. It provides examples of civil society organizations that have promoted budget transparency in several countries, with good results for resource allocation and delivering services efficiently. The chapter concludes by showing how special surveys can obtain public expenditure information even when government financial reporting is weak. Public Expenditure Tracking Surveys from Senegal and Mozambique demonstrate how this information can help diagnose problems in the flow of funds from central governments to service delivery points.

Conclusion

Corruption is a public health issue that will not go away on its own. Fortunately, we can diagnose and prevent it. Rather than responding with despair, shrugging our shoulders, or thinking that it is only a matter for the police to investigate, those of us engaged in public health policy and health-care services should recognize that we can confront corruption by changing the conditions that support it. As the examples in this book show, we can close off opportunities for corruption by creating mechanisms for transparency and ensuring accountability for results. By openly addressing health sector corruption, then, we can come closer to realizing our goal: societies in which everyone has equitable access to health-care services.

References

Azfar, O. 2005. Corruption and the delivery of health and education services. In *Fighting corruption in developing countries: Strategies and analysis*, ed. B.I. Spector, chap. 12. Bloomfield, CT: Kumarian Press.

Emerging Markets Group. 2005. *Armenian reproductive health system review: Structure and system inefficiencies that hinder access to care for rural populations.* Washington, DC: Emerging Markets Group.

Gupta, S., H.R. Davoodi, and E. Tiongson. 2002. Corruption and the provision of health care and education services. In *Governance, corruption and economic performance*, ed. G.T. Abed, and S. Gupta. Washington, DC: International Monetary Fund.

Lewis, M. 2007. Informal payments and the financing of health care in developing and transition countries. *Health Affairs* 26, no. 4:984–97.

Vian, T. 2008. Review of corruption in the health sector: Theory, methods and interventions. *Health Policy and Planning* 23, no. 2:83–94.

World Bank. 2005. *Azerbaijan health sector review note*, vols. I and II. Washington, DC: World Bank.

CHAPTER 2

Fighting Fraud in Hospitals

Stephen N. Musau and Taryn Vian

Hospitals are vulnerable to corruption. In the United States, health-care fraud has been estimated to cost US$60 billion per year, or 3% of total health-care expenditures—much of it in the hospital sector. Hospitals account for 50% or more of health-care spending in many countries. Fraud and corruption in hospitals negatively affect access and quality, as public servants make off with resources that could have been used to reduce out-of-pocket expenditures for patients or improve needed services. This chapter discusses common types of fraud, which occur in hospitals in low-income countries, and suggests ways to prevent and control fraud.

Introduction

According to the National Health Care Anti-Fraud Association in the United States (www.nhcaa.org), health-care fraud is an intentional deception or misrepresentation that could result in unauthorized benefit. In health-care systems that are insurance based, health-care fraud often involves fraudulent reimbursement and billing practices. Within private, for-profit providers and health-care suppliers, fraud may include falsification of financial statements to deceive regulators, shareholders, or industry analysts. Embezzlement, or the misappropriation of property or funds legally entrusted to someone in their formal position as agent or guardian, is another type of fraud.

Hospitals in low-income countries are particularly vulnerable to fraud in part because administrative systems are not well developed or transparent, making it hard to distinguish between intentional fraud, and abuse due to incompetence or ignorance. In addition, hierarchical structures and personnel management systems may discourage people from voicing concerns or pointing out poor performance or irregularities for fear of retaliation.

According to auditors who have worked in resource-constrained hospitals, three types of fraud are particularly common. These include (1) diversion of patient fee revenue at point of service; (2) diversion of accounts receivable, or checks submitted by patients or companies to pay debts owed on their accounts; and (3) collusion between hospital purchasing agents and suppliers. Each of these is discussed below.

Diversion of Fee Revenue

Many hospitals in developing countries charge fees for services. While on average the fee revenue in public hospitals does not often amount to much—generally less than 10% of hospital revenue—it can still be an important source of local funding for essential items such as medicines, supplies, basic maintenance, and small repairs. In private hospitals, fee revenue is the most significant source of funding. Generally, a patient will pay the user fee at a cash collection office, where a clerk records the amount paid and issues a receipt to the patient. There could be several cash collection offices spread across the campus of the hospital, usually close to where services are rendered. At the end of the day, the cashier will prepare a summary of cash collections and deliver this, together with the cash collected, to the accountant (or chief cashier in a large hospital). The accountant or chief cashier will then "post" or record the transactions into the cashbook and into a patient revenue account in the general ledger. The daily cash collections are banked on the next business day by the accountant or chief cashier. In many cases, the accounting function is kept separate from the cash collection function.

One way in which fraud occurs in the process of collecting and recording fee revenue is through the use of a "refund" account. A refund account is an accounting category meant to include revenue to pay legitimate refunds for services that were charged in advance (e.g., a deposit required before a hospital admission) or where a refund is due for some other valid reason. However, refund accounts can also be abused. Instead of posting patient user fee revenue to a patient revenue account, the accountant may post the revenue into a "refund" account. Later, she can make a fictitious "refund" to a nonexistent client, which she actually banks in her own personal account. This type of fraud can be controlled through the introduction of better internal control procedures, such as requiring a higher level of authorization for the release of refunds.

Another way that fee revenue is diverted is by altering receipts. Many government accounting offices and NGOs that lack computers use Kalamazoo-brand manual business supplies such as registers, forms, and receipt books. To avoid the possibility of fraud, it is advisable to fill out receipts with the amount noted in numbers and in words (i.e., "$10.00" and "Ten dollars and no cents"). However, some common types of Kalamazoo receipt books do not have enough space to write the amount of cash received in words. When this information is omitted, it is much easier for someone to change a number on the receipt. In one hospital, an audit detected that cashiers were in fact doing just that. The cashiers would slip a card between the original and the copy so that they could give the patient a receipt for one amount and then, later, go back and fill in a different amount on the carbon copy. The difference between the amount they received from the patient and the lower amount they entered on the carbon copy could be pocketed without anyone knowing. The use of electronic cash registers can help avoid this type of fraud. Another strategy for prevention is to alert patients to watch how the receipt is prepared, and ask them to report any suspicions or concerns.

Diversion of Accounts Receivable

A second type of fraud involves payments for billed services. Many hospitals record the money they are owed as soon as they provide a service in a category called accounts receivable. When patients later come in to settle their debt with a check or companies send a check to pay for services, accounting clerks who receive the checks may deposit them into a personal bank account. Since the debt still appears as owed by the client, the accountant may later write off the client's outstanding balance as "bad debt" or may wait for another check from a different patient/client and apply this to the account whose check was stolen. This is termed lapping, or "teeming and lading." This type of fraud can be avoided by separating duties, that is, having one person open the mail or handle customer cash while a different person is responsible for cash deposits and collection follow-up. Providing monthly statements to clients, and requiring employees to go on leave regularly, can also help expose this kind of fraud.

Collusion With Suppliers

The third major type of fraud in hospitals in developing countries involves collusion with suppliers. After personnel, purchases of goods and services is the next largest expense item. Accountants and purchasing clerks may collude with suppliers to make a deliberate overpayment for an order. The amount by which the order was overpaid is then refunded by the supplier company to the accountant directly, as a kickback. Sometimes a supplier will legitimately offer a "discount" off their list price. In this case, the refund check may be made out to the hospital and will be sent at a later date. In such a situation, the accountant can still commit fraud by depositing the check into his or her own personal account.

Prevention and Control

Improvements in administrative and financial systems can deter employees from attempting these types of fraud. These systems aimed at preventing and controlling fraud are generally part of an organization's internal control system. According to the Committee of Sponsoring Organizations (COSO) of the National Commission on Fraudulent Financial Reporting (also called the Treadway Commission), a system of internal controls "can help an entity achieve its performance and profitability targets, and prevent loss of resources. It can help ensure reliable financial reporting. And it can help ensure that the enterprise complies with laws and regulations, avoiding damage to its reputation and other consequences. In sum, it can help an entity get to where it wants to go, and avoid pitfalls and surprises along the way."[1] The design of an internal control system depends on the size of the organization and the nature of its transactions. Certain aspects of an internal control system may also require investment in staff and/or equipment and hence cost may be a factor to consider in deciding what kinds of controls an organization puts in place. Recommended controls include the following.

Segregation of Duties

The division of duties between cashiers and accountants can help to control against fraud. Where feasible, these two functions should be separate. The cashier is responsible for collecting cash and issuing receipts to patients. The cashier prepares a summary at the end of the day to show how much revenue was received in cash and how much was accounts receivable, payable by patients personally, by employers, or by insurance companies. The cashier's summary should also indicate the sources of the revenue, that is, what service the patient was paying for: laboratory, x-ray, inpatient, outpatient consultations, etc. This allows the hospital to perform a reconciliation report that compares patient volumes from the different service areas with the revenue received.[2]

The accountant's role is to record transactions and he should not handle cash at all. The accountant receives details of cash collected from the cashier and enters them into the accounting records. If the accountant has to handle cash for banking, it is important that the banking records are cross-checked against the cashier's summary by someone more senior—for example, the administrator—to make sure that all cash collected has been banked. None of the cash should be used for "petty cash," or small, discretionary hospital expenditures where it is not feasible to pay by check.

Comparing Actual and Expected Revenue

Another control against fraud is to compute expected revenue and compare it to actual revenue. Health statistics such as patient volumes from each department can be multiplied by the average prices of services to estimate expected revenue per service. When actual cash and accounts receivable are compared with the expected revenue, they should be approximately equal. Gaps should be investigated as they could be due to fraud. This control is not very difficult to implement but requires that at the point of cash collection the source of the revenue is noted (e.g., laboratory, x-ray, inpatient stay, etc.). To enhance the effectiveness of the control, the staff in the department that provides the service could also record in their treatment registers the amount of money that the patient paid or that treatment was on credit. Each department should be required to present a monthly report to the administrator that shows the volume of services rendered and how these services were paid for: cash, accounts receivable, etc. The administrator can then compare the departmental workload and revenue reports with the cashier's revenue report to make sure that they are similar. This was one of the most important controls over revenue in Kenya when user fees were re-introduced in the early 1990s. Other aspects of user fee fraud and general financial performance monitoring are discussed in Chapters 4 and 12.

A possible drawback of this control is that staff in the departments providing services may resist being asked to perform "financial" duties. Careful explanation that they are protecting their service's revenue, and that losses of cash lead to nonavailability of the supplies and tools they need to do their work, may help overcome resistance. The monthly reports they prepare would also show how much their department is contributing to the total revenue of the hospital; any loss of cash reflects badly on their department.

Internal Audit

In low-income settings, some large public hospitals will have an internal audit department that audits payments and other aspects of the financial management system. Where an internal audit function is affordable, this can be a very valuable component of the internal control system, but only if it is given the ability to function independently and without interference from other hospital staff. The internal auditor should report to the chief executive and should be given authority to obtain any documents she may need to examine. The hospital can determine what value of transaction must be internally audited so that the internal auditor need not see each and every transaction. An internal auditor is not restricted to checking the accuracy or authenticity of transactions only but is also involved in checking the functioning of all financial management systems, including internal controls.

Hospitals that cannot afford to hire an internal auditor may choose to have external auditors perform an interim audit (or audits) during the year so that irregularities can be detected before much damage is done. These interim audits form part of the annual audit, increasing the overall cost. NGO hospitals in a network may be able to make the cost of internal audit more affordable by hiring an internal auditor who is shared within the network. However, this may not catch some frauds until after they are committed since this individual would not be fully resident at the hospital. He would, however, be able to do these audits more regularly and frequently than the external auditor and may also reduce the cost of the external audit.

External Audit

The use of competent external auditors, although important, should act as a last defense, since it happens only after 12 months and much damage can be done during that time. In many countries, external audit is a legal requirement for private organizations whether they are for-profit or not. The external audit serves an important role as it allows an independent, technically qualified, registered person to examine the annual financial reports and the underlying accounting records and systems and to issue a report as to whether the financial statements are free of material error. In the process of examining transactions, fraudulent activities can also be detected and reported to management. However, the detection of fraud is not the objective of an external audit.

When evidence of fraud is discovered during an external audit, the auditor is supposed to report it to management. It is up to management to decide whether to hire the external auditor or another financial investigator, to do a special investigation to determine those involved and the extent of the fraud. Management can use the investigator's recommendations for systems improvement and can also use the report to bring legal proceedings against the fraudulent staff.

Investing in Fraud Control: Costs and Sustainability

The internal control systems to prevent fraud need to be tailored to the hospital's size and volume of transactions. Often, relatively small investments in technology can provide major benefits. For example, cash registers can easily reduce the ability of cashiers to tamper with patient fees.

The major cost is the initial purchase of the machines.[3] Use of more sophisticated receipts, which allow more information to be captured, may increase supplies cost only marginally. However, hiring new staff in order to segregate duties may be more difficult to justify. It is important to weigh the benefits of any course of action with the potential cost and decide the best way forward. A good place to start is to look at what improvements a hospital can make with existing resources. Can staff be asked to do new duties that are outside their current job description? Can the hospital form an Internal Controls Team whose duties would be to ensure that the existing controls are being followed? New charts showing side-by-side revenue and volume of services for each department would require little time investment and yet would quickly alert to any major discrepancies.

In addition to investing in information technology and audits, internal controls work best when supported by mechanisms for beneficiaries and employees to raise concerns without fear of retaliation. Complaint boxes are sometimes placed in waiting areas but patients must trust that the information will be read and acted upon confidentially. Making the community aware that they can complain requires outreach to establish this as a channel for getting tips on malfeasance. Facility managers who are trusted members of the community are more likely to be successful. In some cases, they have given out their phone numbers and urged beneficiaries to call anytime.

Employees are another source of information about fraud. A legal framework to protect whistle-blowers is important but so is facility-level policy and leadership. Managers can encourage staff to report suspicions about fraud or ideas for how to strengthen systems to prevent abuse. This input can help to target systems improvements in cost-effective ways, but adequate anonymity and protection must be provided.

Conclusion

Fraud takes place in hospitals if the environment is such that the perpetrator perceives little risk of being caught. This is particularly so if cashiers, accountants, and stores clerks think that nobody is looking at what they do: there is no demand for reports; no comparisons between revenue and service volume reports; no regular checking of service registers or cashbooks. Clearly the involvement of senior management in supportive supervision is important in sending the message that somebody is looking and is ready to take action. Strengthening internal control systems is important and can start with making better use of existing resources before incurring additional costs.

Notes

1. Internal Control–Integrated Framework. Committee of Sponsoring Organizations (COSO) 1992.

2. See Chapter 12 for further discussion of how comparing expected versus actual revenue and expenses can help detect anomalies and deter corruption.

3. See Chapter 4 for more details on the Kenya cash registers initiative.

Further Reading

Biegelman, M.T., and J.T. Bartow. 2006. *Executive roadmap to fraud prevention and internal control: Creating a culture of compliance.* NJ: John Wiley & Sons.

De St. Georges, J.M., and D. Lewis. 2000. How can you protect yourself from employee dishonesty? *Journal of the American Dental Association* 131: 1763–4.

Schulhof, B. 1996. The ABC's of computer embezzlement. *American Journal of Orthodontics and Dentofacial Orthopedics* 110, no. 1:112–3.

Sparrow, M.K. 1998. *Fraud control in the health care industry: Assessing the state of the art.* Washington, DC: National Institute of Justice, U.S. Department of Justice. www.ncjrs.gov/pdffiles1/172841.pdf (accessed August 31, 2009).

Sparrow, M.K. 2008. Fraud in the U.S. health care system: Exposing the vulnerabilities of automated payment systems. *Social Research* 75, no. 4: 1151–80.

Wells, J.T. 2002. Lapping it up. *Journal of Accountancy* (February). www.aicpa.org/pubs/jofa/feb2002/wells.htm (accessed September 1, 2009).

CHAPTER 3

Embezzlement of Donor Funding in Health Projects

Katherine Semrau, Nancy Scott and Taryn Vian

Donor funding has helped to fuel a vast increase in service delivery, medical research, and clinical trials throughout the developing world. Yet, there is a dark side to this badly needed influx of funding. Existing management systems are often weak, and with pressures to spend quickly and achieve results, projects may not pay sufficient attention to internal monitoring and security systems to protect against employee embezzlement. This chapter analyzes how embezzlement can happen in a donor-funded project, and what can be done to prevent or mitigate the risk of such corruption.

Background

Embezzlement is defined as the misappropriation of property or funds legally entrusted to someone in their formal position as an agent or guardian. Everyone wants to believe that the people they have hired are good employees who can be trusted to perform with integrity. Yet, research shows that embezzlement may arise even among the most well-trained, hardworking, and trusted employees in an organization (De St. Georges and Lewis 2000). The scope of corruption and fraud in international aid projects, especially, is frequently underestimated. Berkman (2008) argued this point in his book *The World Bank and the Gods of Lending*, calculating that US$100 million per year was stolen from World Bank–funded projects in Nigeria in the 1990s, mainly because the procedures for disbursement, although rational, depended "completely upon the integrity of those managing the process—and this is where things would fall apart" (p. 77). Abuses include fraud in the form of inflated or fictitious invoices, padded travel expenses, and diversion of project assets to private use.[1]

Donor-funded projects in developing countries are particularly vulnerable to employee fraud for several reasons. First, the nature of project support and short implementation timetables often require large amounts of funds to be spent in a small amount of time. Under pressure to spend quickly, project managers often fail to monitor project expenditures closely or set up appropriate financial checks and balances. Second, donors often need to establish bank accounts in both foreign (hard) and local currencies. While this arrangement may protect against currency risk from inflation, extra accounts add to the complexity of the financial system and make tracking expenditures and transparency more difficult. Third, many everyday transactions needed to implement a field project in poorly developed economies are cash based and vulnerable to theft. Finally, the temptations for employees to be dishonest may be less visible to donor organizations: employees may have credit problems, have a criminal history, or come under pressure from their families to extract resources from employers—all factors that create pressures or motivations to embezzle. Preventing embezzlement, therefore, is linked to strengthening financial systems, selecting financial staff who are less susceptible to pressures and temptations, and implementing supervisory and control systems for early detection of problems.

The project discussed here illustrates one example of how embezzlement occurs. Project ABC is a multiyear research project with a multimillion dollar budget conducted by a US-based NGO in "Belletown," an urban city in eastern Africa.[2] Although the setting is a research project, the story is typical of the causes and consequences of embezzlement in many types of international aid projects.

Project ABC and Its Financial Control System

Project ABC was designed to conduct a clinical trial on a treatment for a common disease prevalent in the region. The project was structured such that project administration and the laboratory were based at the same facility, the central office. Two satellite sites were located at Ministry of Health clinics in Belletown and were staffed by project-funded nurses, counselors, and doctors. These clinic staff were responsible for participant recruitment, all clinical and medical procedures, primary data and specimen collection, and participant follow-up. A subject manager at each clinic was responsible for staff supervision, basic clinic operations, and regular reporting to the project manager based at the central office. The project manager had overall responsibility for Project ABC, including human resources, financial management, and the integrity of the clinical trial. The project manager, a US expatriate posted to Belletown, hired a project administrator to assist with the financial and human resource management. The project administrator's CV indicated that he had previous experience in finance and specific training in financial management.

Typically, Project ABC spent US$15,000–US$20,000 per month in field office costs, including transportation costs incurred by the study partici-pants, medicines, general office costs such as rent and office supplies, and salaries for local staff. Expenditures were made primarily in cash from the central or main office and from satellite offices located at two clinical sites where patients were seen.

Project ABC followed the common procedure of transferring funds from the funding agency to the NGO's US-based head office and then wiring them to a local checking account at an international bank in Bel-letown, where it was kept in foreign (USD) and local (LC) currency. This procedure had the advantage of insulating the funds from the effect of local currency fluctuation until the project staff were ready to make pur-chases. Project staff would then withdraw money from the local US-dollar account in two ways. First, some money was regularly transferred to the LC checking account to pay for salaries, insurance, medicines, rent, and other monthly bills. Second, funds were withdrawn as cash and put into the office safe to be used at the two patient clinics and the head office to pay for day-to-day costs such as transportation reimbursement and for items purchased from vendors who did not accept checks.

A financial software package was used to record expenditures, which were documented largely with paper receipts. Clinic staff tracked subject reimbursements and bonuses, using handwritten ledgers, which were later reconciled at the central office. The subject manager at each satellite site was accountable for reviewing and verifying receipts prior to sending them to the central office. Once receipts were received at the central office, expenditures were reviewed and reconciled by the project administrator. After paper receipt review, another cash allotment was provided to the clinic.

Project ABC staff knew the importance of regular financial reporting, both within and outside the project. The project administrator balanced the bank statements monthly at the central office. The project manager then reviewed them and sent the expenditure reports and electronic files to the US-based office of the NGO. A program manager, based in the United States, was responsible for the final review of the financial reports and reporting the expenditures to the NGO's US office administration and the financial donor institute.

Annual financial audits from the NGO's US office, and the internal monthly and annual reviews, were completed for 3 years without any seri-ous incident. Over time, the expatriate project manager granted complete financial responsibility to Bob, the project administrator. Bob had been working with the project since its inception. He was extremely person-able, respected, and trusted by the management staff both in-country and at the US-based NGO head office. As the project expanded, granting

Bob more responsibilities was a natural progression as he was increasingly considered a valuable employee who contributed significantly in all areas of the project. He accepted the increased responsibility readily and appeared to be adequately managing both the human and financial resources.

Problems Arise

In the spring of 2003, the expatriate project manager left for another position and was replaced. During the transition period, the old and new project managers worked together to review data. While reconciling the cash receipts and cash in the safe, a significant amount of money was noted as missing (LC 5,000,000 or about USD 2,000). When the project managers asked Bob, as the project administrator, about the missing funds, he replied that some receipts might have been accidentally misplaced, but he could not produce them.

The two project managers knew they had a problem and conducted a more in-depth review. They started by examining the expenditures and withdrawals of cash from the bank account over the last 6 months. Graphing cash withdrawals over time, they observed an increasing trend of cash withdrawals from the bank. The amount and frequency of withdrawals had nearly doubled during this period. Furthermore, the overall expenditures in the field office significantly increased during the same period, specifically, the expenditures for fuel, cell phone minutes, and car servicing. After 2 weeks of review, they determined that USD 20,000 was missing. The project managers quickly realized that the most likely cause of the problem was embezzlement and that Bob was most likely responsible.

Diagnosis: Corruption

The problems above—namely, skimming cash from project bank accounts and unauthorized or undocumented expenditures—were related to weak internal controls within Project ABC's financial management system. A review of financial systems showed that the procedures currently in place did not provide adequate protection against fraud by a highly placed employee like Bob. Project ABC's financial system established at project inception had not been revised to accommodate the increase in the volume of transactions as the project developed. Three important controls were inadequate: (1) the system did not include independent verification of the bank statement to computer totals; (2) the system did not provide for adequate segregation of financial duties for checks and balances—thus, it was possible for someone to abuse his or her position for private gain without it being detected by someone else; and (3) the system did not adequately monitor and control transactions or require some transactions to have special approval. The inadequacies of each of these internal controls are detailed below.

Independent Verification of Bank Statements

Good internal control procedures require reconciliation of project accounts to bank statements. Although the project's bank statements were compared with the computerized financial records each month, the dishonest employee was the one mainly responsible for the comparison. Because the project manager trusted Bob, review of his work was not as thorough as it could be. Additionally, at the NGO's US head office, accounts were only being reconciled from the receipts to the computerized financial records but not to the actual withdrawals registered in the bank statements. Bob was able to manipulate the receipts and computer records so that they matched. The reconciliation to the bank statements was the only way to catch the fraud, and no one did this.

Segregation of Financial Duties

The project administrator performed almost all of the financial functions. This is common in a small project. For example, when creating the bank accounts years earlier, the NGO had only requested one signatory due to the small staff size and the difficulty in obtaining double signatures on all checks. However, because of this Bob was able to withdraw, distribute, and account for all project cash. This allowed him to withdraw and pocket cash, without being caught, at least until the change in project management staff created the occasion for a special review. He was also able to purchase cell phone minutes and fuel without proper documentation.

Monitoring and Control of Transactions

Project ABC's financial management system was set up to tightly control expenditure transactions involving lower-level employees and satellite clinics. However, Project ABC did not anticipate the potential for abuse at the managerial level. While the system adequately controlled for study participants' reimbursements and a staff bonus system, the project did not have strong controls or ways to track use of cell phone minutes or out-of-pocket reimbursements for managers. Staff were not required to sign receipts for receiving project-funded resources such as phone cards, and receipts for transactions were simply left on the administrator's desk with no record of who did the purchasing. In addition, the satellite clinic cash was not counted and reconciled with the recorded transactions each day.

Interestingly, later interviews with staff suggested that they were aware of the embezzlement but did not feel it was their role to say something. It appeared that many people, and not just Bob, were benefiting personally because of the weak internal financial controls. In addition, a sense of power imbalance between staff and project management found in many international aid projects, and a lack of mechanisms for safely and anonymously voicing concerns, might have prevented the transgressions from being revealed earlier.

Immediate Actions Are Taken

Once the embezzlement was discovered, the project manager took immediate action to deal with those responsible for the embezzlement, try to recover the money, and report the misappropriation. At the Project ABC, the project manager took immediate control of all financial responsibilities. The NGO also confronted Bob formally, offering him an opportunity to present a legitimate explanation. However, Bob could not produce any clear explanation for the missing money and admitted only that he had failed in his responsibility to adequately manage the funds.

It was clear that Bob could not continue working for the organization, both to prevent further embezzlement and to demonstrate to staff that people would be held accountable for their actions and mismanagement would not be tolerated. However, dismissing a staff member is often difficult even when convincing evidence of wrongdoing is available. In Project ABC, the NGO's human resource policies and national labor laws made it difficult to fire Bob. Instead, the NGO decided not to renew Bob's contract, which, fortunately, was expiring soon. Bob was paid through to the end of his contract and was told not to return to work. For a number of reasons, including the lengthy and uncertain process of filing a criminal complaint, Project ABC opted not to pursue a formal investigation and therefore could not recover the money.

To be fully transparent, Project ABC reported the incident and remedial plan to the CEO of the NGO and to the funding agency. The funding agency did not punish Project ABC or the NGO; however, the reported embezzlement meant that the NGO project no longer qualified for special "expedited financial reviews" by the funding agency. This meant that the annual performance review and budgeting process was now much longer and required more approvals. In addition, the financial offices at the NGO's US head office required additional monitoring and review procedures for the accounting process.

Strategies to Prevent Embezzlement

In moving forward, Project ABC first took steps to discuss what had happened with project staff. Staff had heard rumors of problems, and some had been interviewed in the course of the investigation. Project ABC felt that being transparent about the problem would help employees see that the leadership was fully committed to ensuring accountability and would be proactive about preventing and deterring fraud in the future. The project wanted to begin creating a system of compliance and accountability that would become an integral part of the organization's culture. Changing culture takes time, but the commitment to fraud detection and prevention was seen as an essential step toward promoting ethical behavior.

Second, Project ABC implemented a set of activities to prevent embezzlement in the future, including systems redesigned to strengthen internal control. Project ABC contracted a financial specialist to develop a better financial system. Within 1 month of Bob's dismissal, the new system was in place, with stricter internal controls on cash transactions, segregation of financial duties, and proper steps to reconcile accounting records with bank statements. For example, cash was now kept in the main safe, with only the project manager having the keys, and procedures for weekly cash counts by a minimum of two staff were instituted. A voucher system was implemented with cash reimbursement or advances made only with written authorization from the project manager, after which the administrator made payments. The new vouchers recorded the names and signatures of those who (1) prepared the voucher, (2) authorized the voucher, (3) paid it, and (4) received the cash, again increasing the tracking and accountability of all cash flows. Reconciliation of each voucher with change and formal receipts was required within a week after payment.

A new "imprest" (petty cash) system was also implemented. Each petty cash transaction required a voucher and appropriate receipts and was tracked by category in a simple spreadsheet. When the account was depleted, the financial manager prepared a printed report from this spreadsheet, submitted it to the project manager for authorization, a cash count was conducted, and the account was refilled up to the limit. In another effort to separate financial functions, all major transactions were now paid only by the project manager, with lower level transactions approved by the new financial manager.

The old computer financial software system was reconciled as well as possible given existing records, closed out, and started anew. All vouchers were entered into the software accurately, and electronic files, bank statements, and the paper vouchers were sent to the NGO's US head office to be reviewed again, this time from all angles. Cash counts were conducted weekly by at least two people, to ensure that cash on hand was equivalent to that recorded electronically in the software.

Project ABC immediately removed Bob as a bank account signatory and began requiring two account signatories for every transaction. A short-term administrative consultant was hired to write an organizational financial manual based on recent management policies and decisions. This administrative consultant helped implement the new procedures and ensured that the local staff were adequately trained in all areas of financial management. The project manager and at least one other staff member initiated spot-check audits to check cash balances and vouchers. Additionally, the NGO's US office began to conduct comparisons of the bank statements, paper receipts, and financial reports on a monthly basis. Three years later, the project has not had problems. The NGO now uses the strengthened financial systems as a model for all new projects.

Finally, Project ABC shared the lessons it had learned with other NGOs. Although it was hard at first to overcome embarrassment at having been the victim of embezzlement, Project ABC quickly found that others had experienced similar problems. This confirmed the widespread nature of embezzlement concerns, whether petty or grand. Most NGOs that had experienced fraud reported that they did not prosecute but instead had dismissed the guilty employee as Project ABC had done with Bob. Often, small NGOs are not equipped with the human resource capacity or financial resources necessary to prosecute in a foreign country. Moreover, NGOs are typically subject to the time frame of a donor grant, further constraining their ability to prosecute employees committing fraud. While criminal prosecution of Bob by Project ABC would have been an opportunity to set the precedent to deter NGO fraud and embezzlement, the obstacles to action seemed too great. Policy interventions to support small NGOs in prosecuting suspected guilty employees will be an important step in fighting corruption in international aid work.

Conclusion

The global agenda for development means that aid money is expanding to unprecedented levels. While not widely publicized, many organizations have dealt with the frustrations of financial mismanagement, embezzlement, and theft. The experience of Project ABC suggests several avenues for preventing embezzlement through tighter financial controls, better management policies, and channels for disclosure, all of which increase the likelihood of detection. For projects that are just beginning, establishing a sound financial system and planning for improvements and adjustments of that system over time should be a priority. Even in small projects with limited budgets, simple steps can be taken to strengthen internal financial controls and reduce the risk of employee fraud. While no system is foolproof, changes in policies, procedures, and reporting can help promote a culture of compliance and avoid corruption.

Notes

1. See also Kramer, W.M. 2007. Corruption and fraud in international aid projects. U4 Brief No. 4. www.cmi.no/publications/file/?2752=corruption-and-fraud-in-international-aid-projects.

2. It has been necessary to disguise Project ABC and change details of the case in order to protect the privacy of informants; however, details crucial for interpretation of the nature and consequences of embezzlement have not been changed. While written from the perspective of a donor-funded NGO, the vulnerabilities to embezzlement are universal concerns for local NGOs and local governments as well.

References

Berkman, S. 2008. *The World Bank and the gods of lending.* Sterling, VA: Kumarian Press.

De St. Georges, J.M., and D. Lewis. 2000. How can you protect yourself from employee dishonesty? *Journal of the American Dental Association* 131: 1763–4.

Further Reading

Else, B.C. 1995. Internal control and cash management manual and questionnaires. Technical Report UKR-7. November 1995. Prepared for Polyclinics in Ukraine, under the Zdrav*Reform* Program. www.health.gov.ua/zpr/101-200/0152/0152e.pdf.

KPMG. 1999. *Internal control: A practical guide.* Posted on the European Corporate Governance Institute website, www.ecgi.org/codes/documents/kpmg_internal_control_practical_guide.pdf.

MSH. 2003. Assessing your organization's capacity to manage finances. *The Manager*, vol. 12, no. 2. Boston, MA: Management Sciences for Health. pdf.usaid.gov/pdf_docs/PNACY914.pdf.

CHAPTER 4

Reducing Vulnerabilities to Corruption in User Fee Systems

Taryn Vian

Designed to promote efficiency and expand access to health-care services by leveraging financial contributions from patients, user fee systems are in place in government and private facilities throughout the world. Yet, without proper financial controls and personnel management systems, user fee revenue is vulnerable to corruption. Although typically user fees generate no more than 5–10% of recurrent costs in health facilities and many countries are moving toward abolishing user fees for essential services, these cash transactions provide a temptation to collection staff as well as higher-level government agents.

Perhaps the most typical way that user fees are abused is when a patient pays an official fee for public health-care services, but the fee collector steals the money rather than depositing it in the facility's cash drawer or bank account. In systems with pervasive corruption, fee collectors may be pressured to kickback some of the fees to their supervisors. Exemption systems may also be manipulated, with collection agents exempting individuals (friends or well-connected individuals) who are not entitled to having their fees waived.

This chapter illustrates how the Coast Provincial General Hospital (PGH) in Mombasa, Kenya, tackled the problem of vulnerabilities to corruption and inefficiency in user fee systems.[1] By introducing policy and system changes, Coast PGH was able to reduce corruption, and by instilling responsible stewardship of user fee revenues, it was able to make more funds available for quality improvements.

Situation Facing Coast PGH

Coast PGH in Mombasa is the second largest government hospital in Kenya, with an available bed capacity of 550 and a staff of 660. The primary hospital for the city of Mombasa's population of 600,000, Coast PGH is also the referral hospital for all of Coast Province. The total hospital budget was 3.4 million US dollars[2] in FY1998. About 69.5% was allocated to personnel and 23.4% for nonpersonnel expenditures. Overall, patient fees accounted for 5.7% of total revenue, while reimbursement from the National Hospital Insurance Fund (NHIF) accounted for 1.4%.

In the late 1990s, declining government support for hospital operations, caused by declining GDP growth in the country, made the hospital heavily reliant on cost sharing through user fees to support nonpersonnel requirements. In addition, reimbursements from the NHIF were declining. Total user fee revenue and NHIF billings were about US$243,000 in FY1998, representing about 30% of the hospital's nonpersonnel expenditure budget. Of this amount, about 80% was in cash collections and 20% was insurance billing. Further declines in insurance reimbursement were expected, due to financial difficulties within the National Hospital Insurance Fund.

An assessment of Coast PGH in 1998 concluded that "the existing organizational systems are almost all malfunctioning or broken and need replacement ... dramatic improvements are needed in the organization's performance" (Clark 1999). The report detailed problems in the areas of organization, governance, staffing, patient care, finance, and accounting. Waiting time for patients was very long, and patient satisfaction was low. Patients perceived that service quality was weak and medical personnel had poor manners and negative attitudes. Satisfaction surveys also reported that patients suspected fraud in the revenue-collection process.

On the positive side, during the 1990s, Coast PGH started to receive assistance from the Japan International Cooperation Agency (JICA) to modernize its plant and repair the run-down conditions. The capital improvements were nearing completion in 1998. Additional revenue was needed to support the operation of the renovated facilities. Coast PGH also had strong support from the provincial medical officer, the hospital administrator, and the Hospital Board, all of whom were committed to improving the quality and responsiveness of the hospital.

The Initial User Fee Collection System

Under the cost sharing system in Kenya, government hospitals and health centers could charge nominal fees to patients and seek reimbursement for services rendered to NHIF members. Exemptions existed for certain vulnerable populations and the very poor. Seventy-five percent of the revenues from cost sharing were retained by the facility and spent on nonpersonnel requirements to improve services, and 25% of the revenues were retained at the district level for preventive care measures. User fee revenue was in addition to normal government budgetary allocations, that is, the government budget allocation was not reduced in proportion to revenue collected. Thus, the hospitals and health centers had a positive incentive to collect more user fees.

The administrative system for fee collection covered all the services in the hospital where fees could be charged, that is, outpatient clinics, ancillary services such as the different laboratories and diagnostic equipment centers, and the inpatient billing offices. Collection clerks were stationed in each of these services. For most outpatient services, fees were collected before the client was seen; however, for other services (prescription drugs, for example, and inpatient stays), the cost of services was calculated and paid upon discharge or when the patient visit was over. The clerks collected fees, filling out receipts in triplicate, with one copy kept by the patient, one copy kept by the collection unit, and one copy sent to central accounting. Each clerk also implemented policies for exemptions or waivers of fees for those who qualified. After filling out the receipts, the clerk would put the revenue in a drawer or cash box. At the end of the day or shift, the clerk would write in a ledger book the total cash collected. Supervisors were assigned to collect the cash and review the receipt books, in order to reconcile the information to what was written in the ledger and reported to accounting.

Were User Fees Being Properly Collected?

Coast PGH managers believed that some of their cost sharing revenue was being lost through corruption, but had not done anything about it because they were unsure of its magnitude. Now that they were facing a more serious financial situation, they wanted to raise user fees. Fees were modest when compared with the cost of care and with inflation; however, there was a lack of public confidence in the hospital, and fee increases would not be acceptable to the local community until something was done to decrease fraud and more completely capture the official patient charges.

Part of the user fee collection problem seemed to be collection agents who did not charge their friends, or who charged patients but pocketed the income for themselves. The manual receipt books permitted collection clerks to underreport collections and patients reported that it was difficult to verify their bills. Because of delays and gaps in the data collection and analysis, it was difficult to predict what the user fee revenue was supposed to be.

Plan of Action

The Coast PGH management team began working with consultants to address the vulnerabilities in the user fee system. The first step Coast PGH undertook was to improve the manual system for reporting daily cash receipts. While this strengthened checks and controls to some extent, the manual system was laborious, did not allow daily reconciliation of accounts, and did not provide data quickly enough to verify that the cash collected matched the revenue recorded.

Even with improvements, the manual system could not provide information needed to project expected revenue. Coast PGH managers needed to be able to estimate expected revenue, based on the types and quantities of services provided and standard pricing sheet and exemption criteria, so that they could compare the expected revenue with actual revenue and detect discrepancies. Even with better manual systems, the lack of timely financial information—both estimates of expected revenue and reports of actual revenue by type of service—was still a major obstacle to accountability.

The solution, they decided, was to implement a system of networked cash registers. By implementing the automated cash registers, which would be connected to each other through a local area network, Coast PGH managers could get information on the exact amounts billed, and how much was collected from patients for each type of service. The management team estimated that by implementing the system, they could increase user fee revenues by 25%.

Coast PGH management worked with consultants to develop a detailed request for proposals to implement networked point-of-sale cash registers. Multiple cash collection points were to be reduced to five: Casualty, Outpatient Pharmacy, Laboratory, Maternity, and the NHIF Office. These were linked through a network to a central server in the Accounts Office. After 4 months, through a competitive procurement process, Coast PGH selected an experienced local vendor. The vendor took 3 months to implement the new system, which cost US$42,000 and was paid by the project. It was estimated that the expected increase in annual revenue resulting from the new system would equal or exceed this investment.

The new system operated similar to cash registers in department stores and supermarkets in the private sector in Kenya. After paying her bill, a patient is given a receipt with a printed description of all items paid for, amount paid, and change given. The money received from patients is kept securely in a cash till. The system differed from private sector retail establishments in two important ways: (1) billing for the NHIF was coded into the software and (2) categories were included to account for waivers and exemptions to patients.

The networked cash register system produced several management reports, including daily revenue and cumulative monthly revenue, by fee-for-service item, by cash collection point, by cost center, and by cashier.

Along with software implementation, staff needed to be trained in how to operate the system. Here, the project ran into unexpected problems. Hospital collection staff did not want to attend the training on how to use the new system. In fact, some staff outright refused to be retrained. Coast PGH management, concerned about the potential to undercut the new system, decided to hire new staff who were trained to operate the cash registers. It is possible that existing staff may have resisted the new system because they could see it would constrain their opportunities to pocket user fee revenue.

Results Exceed Expectations

Based on the experience of another hospital in Kenya that had moved to using cash registers, the Coast PGH management team first estimated that cash collections would increase 25%. They collected baseline data on utilization and cash collections for 3 months before implementation, then 3 months afterward, in order to monitor the actual change in revenue. In fact, cash collections exceeded expectations, rising 47.4% (US$24,448 for 3 months prior to implementation to US$36,034 for 3 months after). Despite the substantial increase in revenues, service utilization was unchanged. This suggests that the increase in revenue was almost exclusively the result of reduced theft and not an increase in payments by patients.

Coast PGH management and the consultant team also evaluated staff perceptions regarding the new system. Most personnel were happy with the system and thought it benefited patients. Staff reported no complaints from patients about having to make informal payments to get favors from staff (a practice that some had observed before the system was modified), and there were reportedly fewer complaints about waiting lines, people jumping the queue, or people wandering around to figure out where to make payments.

But implementation was not without problems. Cash register operators complained about irritated eyes and back problems. Some nurses complained that their workload had also increased, possibly from the more rigorous procedures for recording services and supervision. At times, patients were caught giving their used receipts to others to use as evidence of having paid because the receipts did not show the names of patients. Systems were adjusted and staff meetings were held to try to address these problems.

A big advantage of the new system was that the management reports allowed Coast PGH officials to practice continuous quality improvement. For example, after reviewing preliminary results, hospital managers realized that many charges for services were still not being reflected in bills paid at the cash register. With the help of consultants, the management team created a flow chart analysis of the steps for billing and took action to streamline the process. They then reassigned and trained staff so they could implement the new process efficiently. Managers also worked on changing the patient discharge process, improving communication between management and staff, and increasing patient information. The result of all these changes was a further increase in user fee revenue of 36%. The gains achieved through the new system held up over time and revenue collection in FY2001 was 400% greater than that in FY1998.[3]

The unexpectedly large increase in user fee revenues from the new system meant that hospital managers needed to spend money quickly. This, in itself, can be a trigger for corruption, and indeed Coast PGH spending decisions around this time were criticized for lack of transparency, and for allocating resources to low-priority requests. Hospital management responded by introducing more transparency in the planning and budgeting process, to improve accountability.

Conclusion

User fee systems in developing countries are vulnerable to diversion of funds and improper administration of exemption systems for personal advantage. These vulnerabilities can be traced to many causes, including outside financial pressures or social pressure from patients or family members, inadequate supervision, and lack of information with which to monitor performance and hold different organizational units and individual agents responsible. Stronger financial accounting and management information systems can contribute to reducing these vulnerabilities. In large hospitals, the use of networked electronic cash registers can be especially effective in improving accountability, as shown in the case of Coast PGH. More frequent reporting of performance indicators, including expected versus actual cash collection, can help managers detect anomalies, pose questions, explore root causes of problems, and take actions to resolve them.

Networked electronic cash registers are not a foolproof solution. For example, if corruption is pervasive and higher-level managers are colluding with fee collection agents to take funds, technical changes and new accounting systems are not likely to be effective. In addition, if hospital managers lack discretion to discipline staff, resistance to change may hamper the introduction of new financial control systems.

The Coast PGH case study highlights the positive role that outsiders such as consultants or oversight committee members can play in promoting transparency. People inside the system may be too fearful of repercussions to advocate for change, but they may nonetheless support those changes once the issue is raised with external support. While the use of outsiders can help to start the ball rolling, sustained operation of a transparent system requires ongoing management commitment to public service, a difficult and daily challenge.

Notes

1. Information for this brief was obtained through review of project documents and through interviews with consultants who participated in the work described.

2. Prevailing exchange rate was 58 Kenyan Shillings per US dollar.

3. A price increase did take effect in late 1999. Although the changes were modest, this probably contributed to the increase in revenue.

Reference

Clark, J. 1999. Operational assessment of three MoH provincial hospitals (AFS Project, Management Sciences for Health, July 1999), cited in Stover C. *Health financing and reform in Kenya: Lessons from the field. Background document for end-of-project conference for the APHIA Financing and Sustainability Project*, Nairobi, Kenya, May 22–24, 2001.

Further Reading

Collins, D., J. Quick, S. Musau, and D. Kraushaar. 1996. *Health financing reform in Kenya: The fall and rise of cost sharing, 1989–94*. Stubbs Monograph Series Number 1. Boston, MA: Management Sciences for Health (available through the MSH Bookstore at www.msh.org).

Newbrander, W., D. Collins, and L. Gilson. 2000. *Ensuring equal access to health services: User fee systems and the poor*. Boston, MA: Management Sciences for Health (available through the MSH Bookstore at www. msh.org).

Stover, C. 2001. *Health financing and reform in Kenya: Lessons from the field. Background document for end-of-project conference for the APHIA Financing and Sustainability Project*, Nairobi, Kenya, May 22–24, 2001.

PART TWO

Demanding Payment Where Services Should Be Free

CHAPTER 5

Informal Pay and the Quality of Health Care: Lessons From Tanzania

Ottar Mæstad and Aziza Mwisongo

Introduction

Informal payments for health services are common in many transitional and developing countries. Informal payments are often claimed to reduce access to health services, especially among the poorest; however, impacts on the quality of care are less obvious, and both positive and negative consequences are conceivable. This chapter draws on a qualitative study among health workers in Tanzania to describe the nature of informal payments that are taking place in the health sector, and their potential impact on access to and quality of health care. Particular attention is devoted to the policy implications.[1]

Background

Informal payments, defined as cash or in-kind transfers to service providers in excess of official user fees, raise concerns about both access to health care and the quality of the services provided (Transparency International 2006).

In order to gain a better understanding of the practice of informal payments in the Tanzanian health sector, and their potential impact on health service provision, we conducted eight focus group discussions with 58 health workers from one rural and one urban district in Tanzania. Separate group discussions were conducted for each cadre (doctors, nurses, clinical officers, and medical assistants) to stimulate a free expression of experiences and views. Participants represented all the different levels of care (hospitals, health centers, and dispensaries) and included staff from both government and private facilities.

Our findings suggest that patients are making informal payments in order to buy higher-quality services, including shorter waiting times.

Moreover, health workers are involved in "rent seeking" activities, such as creating artificial shortages, in order to extract extra payments from patients. Gifts of appreciation are also common, but the distinction between gifts and bribes is often blurred because apparent gifts may be intended to gain access to better services in the future. Health workers may share the payments received, but only partially, and more rarely within their cadre than across cadres. The discussions revealed that many health workers think that the distribution of informal payments is grossly unfair.

How Informal Payments May Affect Access to Health Services

Informal payments, like formal ones, increase the cost of seeking health services and may therefore induce patients to delay or forego health care. It is therefore argued that informal payments will reduce access to health services, especially for the poor.

This conclusion may, however, be a bit too hasty because local health workers will often be able to differentiate between patients with varying abilities to pay. When such "price discrimination" is possible, health workers may choose to ask poor people to pay only such small amounts as are compatible with their continuing to seek health care. With perfect price discrimination, informal payments do not necessarily lead to a reduction in the utilization of health care. In fact, informal payments may be less detrimental to the poor than formal, and more rigid, user fees.

Our findings suggest, however, that even if health workers were able to discriminate the level of informal payments that people can afford to pay, they might not be interested in doing so. For one thing, taking a small bribe may be just as risky as taking a large one. There may also be social norms that oblige health workers to give a certain minimum level of care to people who have paid a bribe regardless of the amount. In addition, when patients have given a bribe, even a small one, they seem to behave as if they are in a stronger bargaining position vis à vis the health worker and may become quite demanding of the health workers. For such reasons, it may not be worthwhile for a health worker to accept small bribes. Since the poor can offer only small bribes, their access to health services might therefore be reduced.

Another reason why health workers may not want to discriminate on price is that their workload may be too big. Many developing countries have a shortage of health workers, and the use of informal payments may then be a way to ration the demand. The poor are, of course, the most likely ones to reduce their demand. It is not obvious, however, that alternative rationing mechanisms would have been more favorable to the poor.

Finally, even if health workers know which patients are rich and poor, they may not be able to collect informal payments from the rich. People who are better educated are typically more able to claim their rights and thereby resist some of the attempts to collect informal payments. Hence, a system of informal payments may in some cases become more inequitable than formal user fees, because it is only the relatively poor who have to pay.

How Informal Payments May Affect the Quality of Health Services

Our research revealed a variety of mechanisms through which informal payments may affect the quality of health care. A more profound understanding of these mechanisms is of interest because it may improve knowledge of how quality may be reduced or enhanced within a system where informal payments are common practice.

Positive Impacts on Quality

Induce Higher Worker Effort

A positive impact of informal payments on the quality of care is not difficult to imagine when the payment has the character of a fee for service. To provide high-quality services will normally involve some personal (non-pecuniary) costs for the service provider (effort costs). The provider may therefore reduce quality to a minimum unless there is some reward related to high-quality service provision. Such rewards may take many different forms (e.g., satisfaction from helping the patient or from complying with professional quality standards), but for some health workers, monetary rewards may be what is needed in order to persuade them to provide high quality. Informal payments may then induce higher quality of care.

Increase the Effective Supply of Health Workers

When informal payments constitute a large share of the income of health workers, these payments may prevent the workers from taking up alternative or second jobs. Hence, informal payments may increase the total number of health workers and/or increase the total time that each worker is available for service delivery. In a situation with a shortage of health workers, this is likely to improve the quality of the service, both through a reduction of waiting times and through an increase in the time available for each patient. We did not systematically collect data on the amount of informal payments received by the health workers in Tanzania, but examples were reported where clinical officers received more from informal charges than what was on their ordinary salary slip. We have no reason to believe that this is a general pattern, nor can we deny that it is. But there is clearly a possibility that informal payments in Tanzania contribute significantly to keeping up the effective labor supply in the health sector.

Induce Quality Competition Among Health Workers

Although the receivers of informal payments may choose to share what they get with other health workers, our informants suggested that sharing is only partial and does not benefit all. Sharing between workers at different levels of care (doctors and nurses, for instance) appears to be more common than sharing among workers within the same cadre.

Limited sharing of informal payments may in fact have a positive impact on the quality of care, because it creates competition among health workers about becoming the receiver of payments. In essence, the health workers bid for payment by raising service quality, as perceived by the patients.

We would expect the magnitude of this competition effect to depend on the number of caretakers available. A single provider will be in a monopoly situation and no competition will take place. If more workers arrive, the competitive pressure will increase. Hence, in a system where informal payments take place, an additional positive effect on quality may derive from increasing the number of health workers, because of increased competition among the workers for payments.

A quality competition race may lead to a kind of collectively irrational behavior, as seen from the perspective of the health workers. In the extreme case, the health workers may simply be exerting higher effort without being able to extract higher total revenues from their patients. In such cases, norms may develop that induce health workers to compete less aggressively. Statements about health workers who talk condescendingly about colleagues who provide high quality suggest that such norms may have developed in some facilities in Tanzania. In the presence of such norms, the potentially positive effect of competition on service quality is obviously reduced.

Negative Impacts on Quality

Create Artificial Shortages

If there are prospects of receiving informal payments, health workers may be induced to create artificial shortages and thus reduce the quality of the service for those unwilling or unable to pay. For example, if doctors think that patients are willing to pay bribes in order to bypass a queue, there will be an incentive for the doctors to create a queue, for instance by working more slowly. Such activity will increase waiting times, which represents a reduction in the quality of the service.

Another example: Imagine a ward with few health workers relative to the number of patients, implying that patients may be "competing" for the scarce time of the health workers. By reducing the time available for patient care (e.g., by having longer breaks), the patients' willingness to pay for the providers' time may increase at the margin. The "market clearing" price will then increase, which may possibly increase total incomes for the providers, in the same way that a monopolist may benefit from supplying a low quantity since the price per unit will then be higher.

A common strategy, as reported by our informants, is to pretend shortages of drugs and supplies and ask for money from the patients in order to "buy" the missing supplies in the private market. Having received the money, the health worker simply picks the supplies from the available stock at the facility. These strategies can work only because patients think that being "out-of-stock" is common and they see that patients who do not pay are not served. Quality reductions for those who pay bribes are related to the wastage of the providers' time to convince patients of the need to pay, whereas those who do not pay bribes have received incomplete care.

Bargain for a Higher Share of Payments

Health workers may reduce the level of quality in order to bargain for a larger share of what their colleagues have received. One example is when nurses withhold quality in order to put pressure on a doctor to share the bribes that she or he has received. Doctors will often depend on nurses in providing the services required to satisfy the patient. A nurse who suspects that the doctor has received a bribe, without sharing with the nurse, may then start to withdraw care from the patient. A doctor who feels obliged to satisfy the patient will then be forced to reveal that he has been bribed.

Signal That the Threshold Quality Is Low

When informal payments can be extracted, there may be incentives for health workers to reduce the quality of care in order to signal that there is much to gain from paying. Health workers will normally be guided by some professional or ethical standards to provide a certain "threshold" level of services even without any payments. Patients will then be willing to pay only for the value of services beyond the threshold. The problem, of course, is that patients have limited information about the actual thresh-old. Therefore, if a health worker is able to convince the patients that the threshold is low, the patients may become willing to pay more in order to receive a given level of service. One way of signalling that the threshold is low is to provide low quality in the initial stages of a consultation (e.g., to receive the patient in an unfriendly manner, to proceed very slowly with the work, etc.).

Create Frustrations

When a system of informal payments becomes institutionalized to the degree that health workers feel they have a claim to a certain share of the payments, perceived unfairness in the actual allocation of the revenue may in itself impact on the quality of services. Our informants suggested that health workers in Tanzania may feel that they have such claims and that failure to meet their expectations is creating frustration and lower levels of motivation. It is not obvious that such frustration will lead to lower levels of care, but it is not unlikely, and our findings clearly point in this direction.

Signal of Noncorrupt Behavior

In a system where high-quality service is taken as a signal that bribes have been received, noncorrupt health workers may be induced to reduce their quality of care. Our results point in the direction that provision of high-quality care may easily create suspicions about corruption. When this is the case, noncorrupt persons who also want to maintain a high level of self-respect will be discouraged from providing their "normal" level of care. At the same time, of course, the fact that high quality is associated with bribery indicates that it has a positive effect on the quality of services delivered by corrupt health workers. The net effect will, in this case, depend on the relative shares of corrupt and noncorrupt workers. Note that a noncorrupt health worker will experience lower welfare when working in an institution where corruption is prevalent, because he is bound to compromise in one way or another. We might therefore expect noncorrupt workers to seek to move away from these institutions. This might be one explanation why participants in the focus groups maintained that the level of corruption differs across facilities.

Policy Implications

Our findings have potential implications both for policies aiming at a reduction or elimination of practices of informal payment and for policies with the more parsimonious goal of minimizing the adverse effects of informal payments on access to and quality of care. It is important to stress, though, that our limited data do not enable us to make any specific policy recommendations.

1. **Compensate for loss of informal payments in order to keep up the health workforce**

   Since informal payments for some health workers may constitute a significant share of their total income, there is a risk that a sharp reduction in informal payments may reduce the availability of health workers, unless the removal of informal pay is compensated by higher salaries.

2. **Inform communities about resource availability**

   While a general recommendation for reducing corrupt practices would be to increase the supply of scarce resources, our findings suggest that more may be needed. In particular, to increase the supply of drugs may only lead to more money going into the pockets of health workers unless patients are informed that supplies have been increased. Embezzlement related to drug supply can continue as long as patients believe that there is a shortage. Information to patients about resource availability may thus be a key component of anticorruption campaigns.

3. **Increase the number of health workers**

   Increasing the number of health workers may be beneficial by helping reduce the length of queues. This, in turn, reduces opportunities to extract bribes from patients willing to pay to be seen quicker. In addition, increasing the number of health workers could increase the quality of care if it encouraged workers to compete more strongly to obtain the payments from patients who are willing to pay informal fees for better service.

4. **Improve management systems**

   Our participants noted that part of the reason for there being less corruption in some facilities is better systems of supervision and management, which may imply that effective corruption control can actually be achieved in a Tanzanian context through systemic reform. Supervision and management may not, however, be the full explanation for the observation that some facilities have much lower levels of corruption than others. The differences between facilities may reflect that health workers who are non-corrupt seek to come together in facilities with other workers of the same type (self-selection) or that some institutions may have more carefully selected their workers from the pool of noncorrupt workers.

5. **Make punishments for bribery sensitive to the size of the bribe**

As for the debate about informal payments versus formal user fees, our analysis emphasizes that there are inherent distributional problems with a system of informal payments, because (1) scarce resources may tend to be allocated to rich patients rather than to the most needy and (2) health workers may be unwilling to serve poorer people who can only pay smaller bribes because the risks or costs to the worker are just as great as accepting a larger bribe. Policies that punish bribery in proportion to the size of the bribe could offset this distributional tendency by balancing the risks and rewards of accepting different size informal payments. Policies that punish larger bribes more than proportionally could even make health workers be more responsive to those who can only pay small informal payments—but at the risk of legitimating small bribes and excluding the poorest who cannot pay at all.

6. **Stimulate open discussion about the unfairness of the system**

One way to improve quality, if the system of informal payments is accepted, is for personnel in charge of health facilities to initiate discussions with employees about the perceived unfairness in the system. Our findings suggest that if managers reduced the level of frustration by encouraging a fair allocation of informal payments, this could improve morale and quality of care. Such an approach, however, is very risky. Openly discussing the systems of informal payment might undesirably give increased legitimacy to these practices. Moreover, it could also strengthen cooperation among health workers in extracting rents from patients, which in turn could reduce quality of care.

In a well-functioning health-care system, there will be legitimate managerial and social mechanisms in place to induce effort and increase quality services; therefore, informal payments will have little or no potential social value. The question facing poorly functioning health-care systems such as the one in Tanzania is whether there are practical ways to manage informal payments without conceding them any legitimacy. If so, as discussed here, there may be ways to mitigate their detrimental effects on quality of care and take advantage of the few positive effects they may have. However, the corrosive impact of informal payments on the social fabric may be so significant that it may be better to confront the problem directly and fight any form of corruption in the patient–provider relationship.

Note

1. For more about this research, see Stringhini, S., S. Thomas, P. Bidwell, T. Mtui, and A. Mwisongo. 2009. Understanding informal payments in health care: Motivation of health care workers in Tanzania. *Human Resources for Health* 7:53. www.human-resources-health.com/content/7/1/53.

Reference

Transparency International, 2006. *Global corruption report 2006: Special focus: Corruption and health.* London and Ann Arbor, MI: Pluto Press.

CHAPTER 6

Strategies for Reducing Informal Payments

Kelly Miller and Taryn Vian

Introduction

Throughout the world, informal payments for health-care services undermine public policies aimed at assuring equitable and low-cost access to care. Many government health-care systems guarantee citizens' access to a predefined package of services, either free of charge or for a small fee. Yet, despite official policies, health-care providers sometimes demand—or patients offer—to make informal or illegal payments outside official channels. Studies have shown that these payments increase the cost of care to patients, especially the poor, and dissuade some people from seeking care at all.

This chapter explores factors that promote or inhibit the practice of informal payments for health services, and discusses implications for health system governance and performance. Innovative attempts to reduce informal payments are analyzed, including experiences from Albania, Kyrgyz Republic, Cambodia, and Armenia. These cases show that it is possible to reduce informal payments through interventions that address the institutional and social causes of the practice.

Types of Informal Payments

Ensor (2004) developed a typology to categorize three reasons unofficial payments occur in resource-constrained economies (Table 6.1). We have modified this typology to include a fourth category of informal payments: gifts.

The first type of informal payment is a cost contribution given by patients toward care, which has been underfunded by the government. Payments such as these are meant to close the "budget–cost gap." Providers may accept them reluctantly from patients who offer the payments willingly, recognizing that personnel are not being paid a living wage or facilities have not been given an adequate budget to perform the expected

Table 6.1 Types of informal payments

TYPE OF INFORMAL PAYMENT	ILLUSTRATIVE QUOTES FROM PATIENTS
Contribution to care	*The doctor must feed himself.*
	They need money to pay their children's school.
Additional services	*You need to send olive oil to the doctor's house, because this way you can receive better service.*
	The timing of the payment influences the quality and speeds it up.
Abuse of power	*Nurses don't clean your wound if you don't pay them.*
	There have been cases in which doctors say that a pregnant woman needs to be operated even though that is not true. They invent reasons to have an operation.
Gifts	*We are really happy when the baby is a boy, and it is because of this feeling that we give money to the person who makes the announcement.*

Source: Based on data collected by Vian et al. (2004).

services. The second type of informal payment is a way of obtaining additional services beyond the "essential package" guaranteed by government. A patient might offer a payment to avoid having to wait in a long line, or to obtain extra amenities such as a single room. A third type of informal payment reflects misuse of power by providers in order to enrich themselves. Such abuses of power occur when, for example, health workers refuse to treat a patient unless the payment is made. This type of informal payment is certainly of greatest concern for its impact on efficiency, equity, and health outcomes. Finally, the fourth type is a gift, freely given by a grateful patient and, presumably, without creating substantial financial hardship.

This final factor complicates discussions about informal payments because of the difficulty in distinguishing between payments that are compelled and those that are truly voluntary. Indirect communication and social interactions can contribute to confusion over intentions and expectations in patient–provider transactions. Providers might accept a payment because they do not want to insult patients who have intended the payment as a gift. In many countries, people do not see gifts as a problem, because they are usually given after the health-care service was obtained and are voluntary expressions of gratitude.

In practice, it is difficult to classify informal payments because even in cases of blatant extortion, individuals find ways to justify their actions. For example, health workers who are abusing their power to extract payments from patients may rationalize their behavior by calling the payments "gifts." Assessing the character and implications of informal payments requires examining people's explanations for the practice in light of alternative explanations, and reviewing data on ability to pay, health worker incomes, and other contextual factors.

Factors Associated With Informal Payments

Informal payments thrive in countries where governments have under-funded services relative to the benefits promised to citizens. They are common in countries where managers are scarce or poorly trained to provide adequate supervision, or where there are confusing rules about entitlements and patients are not sure about their rights. Informal payments are common in hospitals, but they also occur in primary care settings. They are more frequent in settings where patients feel they have few choices or care options, and where disciplinary actions for illegal or improper behavior are unlikely to be taken (Lewis 2007).

Strategies to Reduce Informal Payments

Acknowledging and Addressing Deficiencies in Government Health Expenditures

Informal payments are driven in part by the imbalance between entitle-ments and available resources. Public policies to resolve the imbalance through changes in entitlements or increases in health expenditures can help reduce informal payment (Gaal et al. 2006).

Increasing Provider Remuneration

Since low salaries often motivate providers to demand or accept informal payments, strategies to address this problem may reduce the practice. Link-ing bonuses to performance can also motivate staff to provide better care.

Formalizing User Fees

Replacing informal payments with a formal fee schedule may be a solution. Revenue retained by facilities can be used to supplement salaries and increase quality of care, resulting in greater patient satisfaction and overall use of services (Akashi et al. 2004).

Enforcing Rules and Punishing Offenders

Prohibiting informal payments can be an effective strategy to deter abuses if the rules are enforced and there are consequences for noncompliance.

Increasing Transparency and Accountability

Clear policies, patient information, and channels for complaints can help to reduce informal payments. This includes making sure that patients are aware of the official fee schedule, know what staff are paid, and understand the policies against informal payments. Facilities should have a means for allowing patients to ask questions or report abuses. Facility governance structures such as hospital boards can also increase accountability and help to deter the practice.

Behavior Change

In cases where patients continue to pay informally when it is not necessary, public policy can directly try to change these behaviors by convincing patients that they will not suffer poorer quality or be "punished" by providers if they refuse to make informal payments. Addressing patients' fears and beliefs must occur within an environment that is actively employing other, visible strategies to eliminate informal payments, such as increasing compensation levels so personnel are paid a living wage.

Examples from Albania, Kyrgyz Republic, Cambodia, and Armenia show how some of these strategies have successfully reduced informal payments in the health sector.

Two Hospitals in Albania

Albania, with a population of 3.6 million and per capita income of US$3,740, is one of the poorest countries in Europe. In 2003, despite the country's stated policy of providing most health-care services free of charge, informal payments to medical personnel were common. Studies suggested that 60–87% of Albanian citizens made informal payments to hospital doctors in order to receive services, and out-of-pocket expenditures accounted for more than 70% of total health expenditures, a percentage higher than that for most other Balkan countries.

Factors influencing informal payments in Albania included low salaries of health staff, a belief that health is extremely important and worth any price, desire to get better quality care, fear of being denied treatment or missing the opportunity to get the best outcome possible, and the tradition of giving a gift to express gratitude. Some other reasons given for the rising prevalence of informal payments were the lack of deterrents, social norms influencing providers, and the growth of capitalistic values in Albanian society.

Tirana Maternity Hospital Formalized User Fees and Increased Transparency

Like many other hospitals in Albania, the 300-bed Tirana Maternity Hospital, a public facility located in the capital city, had problems with informal payments. The hospital director decided to attack the problem, starting in the Wellness Center, an outpatient clinic, which saw 10,000 patients per year. The hospital director knew that he could not fight the problem without doing something about doctors' wages, so he began to strengthen the existing system of officially allowed user fees for drugs and ancillary services (pap smear, mammography, and other diagnostic tests). Working with key staff, the hospital director posted the official fee schedule and streamlined systems for cash receipts, cash management, financial accounting, and reporting.

Through these actions, he was able to increase revenue from 900,000 Leks (US$7,031) to 2,590,000 Leks (US$20,234) over 2 years. This revenue was allocated for staff salary supplements (70%) and for supplies replenishment (30%). The changes had the effect of quadrupling doctors' compensation; auxiliary staff salaries doubled and administrative staff received supplements too. The hospital director also posted signs with his cell phone number, saying no one should make any payments outside the regular channels and if they were asked to, they should call him directly. To reinforce this message, the hospital surveyed patients, using an exit interview and placed suggestion boxes in patient areas to solicit feedback. Utilization at the hospital began to rise, which the director attributed to the center's new policies to reduce informal payments (Vian 2003).

The experience in Tirana Maternity is instructive, yet more must be done to evaluate this type of intervention. For example, comparative analyses to other Albanian hospitals could help determine the effectiveness of the Tirana Maternity Hospital's strategies. One would hope to see lower reported rates of informal payments among Tirana Maternity patients, compared to patients served at other hospitals in the city.

Poliklinika Lui Paster Introduced Performance-Based Compensation and Greater Transparency

Poliklinika Lui Paster is a private clinic offering cancer treatment on a fee-for-service basis. Doctors receive a base salary, plus a payment based on the number of treatments the doctor performs. In 2003, total compensation for doctors averaged between US$800 and US$1,200 per month, compared to public salaries of US$100–US$300 per month. In the first year of the clinic's operation, patients tried to make informal payments or gifts to doctors, even with an official fee schedule. The clinic director posted signs stating that informal payments were not allowed, and kept explaining the system. Over time, the director reported that patients began to understand and accepted that the clinic was serious about not wanting any payments, even gifts, to be made outside official channels.

The initial reluctance of patients to pay only the posted fees shows how difficult it is to change attitudes in a culture where informal payments are prevalent. The clinic director's consistent and continuous explanations of the new system show that changing attitudes and behaviors is a gradual process but can be achieved. Poliklinika Lui Paster successfully combined an incentive-based payment schedule and dedicated enforcement to combat informal payments.

The Kyrgyz Health Sector Reform Formalized User Fees, Changed Payment Systems and Increased Transparency

Following independence from the former Soviet Union in 1991, Kyrgyzstan struggled to transition from a planned to market-led economy. Government expenditures dropped in response to the economic transition, reducing public spending on health care and leading to increased patient contributions. Because of the scarcity of resources and budget constraints, patients were being asked to pay for medical supplies and drugs, which should have been free or included in copayments, and even to make payments to subsidize providers' salaries. Informal payments were also collected for admission to a particular hospital, or for admission without referral, and for nonmedical supplies (sheets, lightbulbs) and for food (Baschieri and Falkingham 2006; Jakab 2006).

Informal payments were one of many problems facing the Ministry of Health (MOH) in 1994 when it began a health sector reform that created a Mandatory Health Insurance Fund (MHIF). In 2001, the government went further, introducing a Single Payer Reform (SPR) that addressed the key reasons people were making informal payments: low pay and confusing entitlements. The SPR clearly defined a specific free care benefits package and a formal copayment schedule for hospital referrals, allowing hospitals to retain copayments and use them to supplement salaries (20%) and pay for medicines and patient food (80%). By introducing a clear system of payments to providers, allowing copayments to be retained by hospitals, and increasing the transparency of the system, the designers of the reform expected that funding would be improved and informal payments reduced.

In 2004, after 3 years of implementation, the reform was declared a qualified success. An evaluation found that an increased percentage of people seeking care at the primary level received receipts and fewer respondents reported giving a gift to health personnel, while in hospitals the proportion of patients that reported making payments for medicines, laboratory tests, and other supplies decreased. At least half of all inpatients did not pay more than they should have according to the fee schedules (Baschieri and Falkingham 2006).

But the reform experienced challenges as well. The evaluation found that the proportion of all patients who reported paying for primary care (which should have been free) rose from 10% to 17% between 2001 and 2004. In hospitals, an increased proportion of families were helping with administering injections, and despite decreased proportions of inpatient contributions for some services, the paying proportions remain high (70% for medicines, 39% for laboratory tests, and 47% for other supplies). Also, even though some health professionals "discount" informal payments charged to the poor, the expenditure still represents a greater share of their total household resources than the informal payments paid by wealthier patients.

More recently, reformers have noticed an increase in incorrect charging of copayments, with recorded revenue being less than what patients reported paying, which in turn was less than the expected patient revenue (based on copayment price times quantity of services provided). These findings highlight the importance of monitoring payment systems to identify weaknesses, as people find new ways to manipulate the system for private gain.

A Cambodian Hospital Formalizes Fees and Addresses Enforcement

Cambodia had a deeply rooted system of corruption in its health sector. Pay was low and civil servants relied on coping strategies such as demanding informal payments or working second jobs in the private sector. Informal payments were so high that in 1999, out-of-pocket spending was 20 times higher than government health expenditure, representing 82% of total health expenditures (World Bank 1999). The Cambodian MOH has tried to improve health-care access and rationalize health-care financing with a National Health Coverage Plan, referral networks, and a National Charter on Health Financing. The National Charter introduced official user fees while supplementing staff salaries and creating incentives for expanded provision of care.

The Takeo Provincial Referral Hospital took part in these reforms with success. In 1996, monthly under-the-table revenue at 176-bed Takeo Provincial Hospital was estimated at US$13,750, more than five times the monthly hospital payroll and 45% of total monthly revenue. Unpredictable public funding, low salaries, few sanctions for misconduct, and no rewards for individual initiative all created systemic problems in resource management and informal payments posed a significant barrier to care-seeking behavior (Barber et al. 2004).

To address these problems, a new financing scheme based on a transparent and official fee schedule was introduced in 1997. Inpatient fees represented 65% or less of previous inpatient informal payments and an exemption process identified patients who should not have to pay. The formal fee schedule was intended to increase utilization and regain public confidence in the health system by assuring predictability and reducing provider subjectivity in assessing payment due. Increased utilization would benefit providers, because bonuses would be linked to volume of hospital activity.

After 1 year of the financing reform, data from patients showed that they were paying less than they had paid before the reforms were introduced. In other words, formal fees had replaced informal fees and were not an additional financial burden to patients. In part because of the lower official fees, utilization levels increased by more than 50% for inpatient and surgical services. Performance-based salary supplements were comparable to the previously received average revenue from informal payments. By 2001, Takeo Hospital was able to phase out external donor support as central government funding and official user fee revenue continued to increase over time. Similar reforms were accomplished in Cambodia's National Maternal and Child Health Center in Phnom Penh, demonstrating that formalizing user fees and implementing organizational change have the potential to drastically improve hospital utilization and equity (Akashi et al. 2004).

Armenia's Maternity Care Voucher Program to Reduce Informal Payments

Armenia has one of the highest reported rates of out-of-pocket health expenditures among its neighbors, averaging 26% of reported household income for the poorest population quintile in 2006 (Primary Healthcare Reform Project 2008). Many of these out-of-pocket payments are informal and are being used to pay for services that should be free under the government's Basic Benefit Package (BBP).

Maternity care, including deliveries and pre- and postnatal care, has been part of the BBP guaranteed to all Armenian citizens at no charge.

However, due to low levels of government funding in the hospital sector, formal and informal payments for maternity services had become widespread. Even for the poor, who are guaranteed a more extensive medical benefit package, out-of-pocket expenses for deliveries were common.

An assessment of structure and system inefficiencies in the Armenian health sector suggested that OB/GYN services reap the greatest amount of informal payments (Emerging Markets Group 2005). It was reportedly common for physicians to pay the head physician a portion of all informal payments collected, thus creating a pyramid scheme within facilities that extended up the chain. Emerging Markets Group also found that while the amount of the informal payment varied from person to person, the practice was institutionalized to the extent that patients were quoted an informal amount as part of a consultation prior to service delivery. They found that patients paid informal payments directly to the physicians, nurses, and even janitors. Patients often had to purchase medicines separately, and it was common practice for family members to have to pay additional fees to visit patients.

In 2008, the Armenian government decided to reduce informal payments and assure that all women have access to free, good-quality services for delivery by introducing a new program of maternity care vouchers. Under the program, pregnant women are issued certificates that they present to providers in return for full coverage of delivery, including medicines and testing.

When a facility is reimbursed for a maternity care voucher, a portion of the funds is shared among staff (approximately 60–65%), while the rest supports medicines and supplies. In tandem with the implementation of the voucher system, obstetricians' salaries were increased modestly, and they were to receive a share of the facility's reimbursement revenue based on volume of services provided.

The MOH displayed posters in every facility and made significant efforts to inform the public of the policy change. In addition, efforts were made to enforce the "no additional charges" requirement by punishing staff who are caught accepting informal payments. In some parts of the country, civil society organizations received grant assistance to promote transparency and government accountability in relation to the certificate system, actively disseminate information about the program, and monitor its implementation.

This is an innovative effort to address informal payments by influencing all the incentives facing providers—including the fees they receive and the scrutiny they are under. The program increases incentives for honest behavior by increasing salaries and linking facility-level reimbursement rates to number of services delivered (so that "funding follows patients"). It also increases the probability of detection by supporting government- and community-based monitoring and enforces administrative laws against public employees who are caught accepting bribes or illegal payments. The initiative provided an opportunity to test the ability of radical shifts in financing, and greater transparency and accountability, to effectively end under-the-table payments.

So far, anecdotal evidence suggests that the program has had a positive impact and has decreased out-of-pocket costs, both formal and informal, paid by patients. However, the government is still concerned about whether the reimbursements made to facilities will be shared equitably with individual clinicians, and whether the increased payments will be enough to deter the practice of informal payments. In addition to ongoing monitoring by the MOH, an external evaluation is planned to assess the success of the program.

Conclusion

Formalizing fees is one of the most common strategies for reducing informal payments and can be effective as demonstrated by cases in Albania, Kyrgyz Republic, and Cambodia. This strategy increased facility revenues that in turn supplemented staff salaries, replenished supplies, and helped phase out donor support. Formalizing fees also increased utilization—in some cases by increasing the predictability of fees and reestablishing public confidence, in other cases by reducing the overall cost to patients.

While formalizing fees can successfully combat informal payments, it does not necessarily address the needs of a country's most vulnerable groups unless the reform also includes some mechanism to exempt or subsidize the poor. To be successful, it appears that formalizing fees also requires a strong public education component, explicitly instructing patients about the services to which they are entitled and that payments in excess of the formal fee schedule are not permitted. Such transparency is a powerful weapon against informal payments, but patients have to be given the opportunity to exercise this power. Finally, if salaries from formal fees are not comparable to what providers were earning from informal payments, they may be tempted to cheat the system and revert to clinician-mediated services that are unnecessarily costly to patients.

Changing behaviors of patients can be a particular challenge even when resources are not a problem. Even in a private clinic that wanted to operate formally, the prevailing norms led people to think they needed to offer informal payments. The director of the Poliklinika Lui Paster in Albania showed that it is possible to modify these norms, but only with strong efforts to educate patients and persistence in enforcing standards.

When governments have the resources to pay for free care, increasing transparency can be an effective policy for confronting informal payments, as the Armenian Maternity Voucher Program shows. Consistent funding from committed sources can help prevent financial burdens from being passed on to patients. Linking bonuses to volume of activity or facility-level reimbursement rates to number of services delivered are also viable alternatives, which may increase provider motivation and reduce reliance on informal payments.

Reducing informal payments is essential to ensure access to affordable, high-quality health-care services. Analyzing factors which cause informal payments and adapting strategies which have worked in other countries to address these factors can help strengthen accountability in the public sector and promote better health for all citizens.

References

Akashi, H., T. Yamada, E. Huot, K. Kanal, and T. Sugimoto. 2004. User fees at a public hospital in Cambodia: Effects on hospital performance and provider attitudes. *Social Science and Medicine* 58:553–64.

Barber, S., F. Bonnet, and H. Bekedam. 2004. Formalizing under-the-table payments to control out-of-pocket hospital expenditures in Cambodia. *Health Policy and Planning* 19:199–208.

Baschieri, A., and J. Falkingham. 2006. Formalizing informal payment: The progress of health reform in Kyrgyzstan. *Central Asian Survey* 25, no. 4:441–60.

Emerging Markets Group. 2005. *Armenian reproductive health system review: Structure and system inefficiencies that hinder access to care for rural populations.* Washington, DC: Emerging Markets Group for USAID.

Ensor, T. 2004. Informal payments for health care in transition economies. *Social Science and Medicine* 58, no. 2:237–46.

Gaal, P., P. Belli, M. McKee, and M. Szocska. 2006. Informal payments for health care: Definitions, distinctions, and dilemmas. *Journal of Health Politics, Policy and Law* 31:251–93.

Jakab, M. 2006. Informal payments in Kyrgyz hospitals: Is informal payment pro-poor? Presentation at the Center for International Health and Development, Boston, MA, May 2.

Lewis, M. 2007. Informal payments and the financing of health care in developing and transition countries. *Health Affairs* 26:984–97.

Primary Healthcare Reform Project. 2008. How great is the burden of household health expenditure in Armenia. Yerevan, Armenia: Emerging Markets Group, PHRP.

Vian, T. 2003. Corruption in the health sector in Albania. *Report prepared for the Albania Civil Society Corruption Reduction Project, Management Systems International for USAID/Tirana.* Boston, MA: Boston University School of Public Health.

Vian, T., K. Gryboski, Z. Sinoimeri, and R.H. Clifford. 2004. *Informal payments in the public health sector in Albania: A qualitative study.* Bethesda, MD: Partners for Health Reform*plus* Project, Abt Associates Inc.

World Bank. 1999. *Cambodia Public Expenditure Review. Poverty Reduction and Economic Management Sector Unit Report 18791-KH.* Washington, DC: World Bank.

PART THREE

Manipulating Procurement and Drug Supply

CHAPTER 7

Pay for Honesty? Lessons on Wages and Corruption from Public Hospitals[1]

William D. Savedoff

Introduction

Theft, kickbacks, absenteeism, and soliciting bribes in the health sector in developing countries are often blamed on low pay. But does low pay actually explain corruption? Several studies of public hospitals in Latin America suggest otherwise. In particular, they show that low pay may contribute to corruption; however, without some form of monitoring to detect corruption and a real chance of penalties, raising wages is not likely to make a difference.

Pay Levels and Corruption

The idea that low pay explains corruption is widespread and seems reasonable (Ferrinho et al. 2004). If someone is poorly paid, the temptation to steal or commit fraud would be greater. However, this does not explain why corruption occurs among well-paid individuals or why so many individuals who are poorly paid remain honest. Whether poorly paid or not, other factors are either more important or necessary for individuals to resort to illicit forms of enrichment. These other factors include the expected gain from corruption, the probability of being detected, and the magnitude of the penalty if caught.

Although low pay is often blamed for corruption, few studies even look at whether civil servants are indeed underpaid. Sometimes the results are surprising. A study in Indonesia, using 1997 data, found that, on average, public sector workers were paid more than their private sector counterparts, with wages that were the same or up to 30% higher (Filmer and Lindauer 2001). The difference was significant for workers with primary and secondary schooling but wages were indistinguishable between public and private sector workers with higher education. This is one way in which the general argument that low pay explains corruption might lack substantiation.

Is Impunity to Blame?

One of the most important ways that pay can deter corruption is if it increases the penalty of being caught and dismissed. If an individual earns a premium in their job above what they would otherwise earn in another job, then that premium is at risk if that individual should commit fraud and be caught and dismissed. One study specifically estimated this premium for purchasing managers at 33 hospitals in the city of Buenos Aires at a time when purchasing was decentralized to each hospital's purchasing department (1996–1997). Similar to the findings in Indonesia, these workers were earning more in their public sector job than they would have elsewhere. The average monthly salary of a purchasing manager was US$1,295, estimated to be about US$375 more than that same manager would earn in another job based on his or her age and experience. Was the risk of losing this premium sufficient to deter corruption?

In this particular case, the concern was that purchasing managers might be soliciting kickbacks, that is, using their positions to inflate the prices paid for supplies in return for receiving a share of the difference; or accepting bribes in order to steer contracts to particular suppliers with higher prices. The study analyzed data on prices paid for nonpharmaceutical medical supplies by Buenos Aires hospitals and the authors argued that the unexplained differences in prices paid across hospitals provided a good indicator of the level of corruption—kickbacks and bribes—in those same hospitals (see Chapter 9 for more detail on the measures and how they were collected). Using this information, the authors tried to see if the premium paid to purchase managers above what they would otherwise earn in the labor market could explain the different levels of corruption. Surprisingly, there was no statistical relationship between pay and corruption—even after making adjustments for hospital size, experience, and other factors.

The study considered several explanations. They rejected the suggestion that there was no corruption in the hospitals based on several surveys and numerous interviews with patients, hospital staff, and administrators (see Figure 7.1). They also rejected the possibility that purchase managers were unresponsive to financial incentives—this is contradicted by a great deal of empirical evidence. Instead, they argued that the size of the earnings premium was unrelated to corruption because purchase managers were under very little risk of losing their jobs. In fact, no purchase manager was ever fired, disciplined, or even investigated during a period when the city's Health Secretariat was collecting the price data that demonstrated large deviations from market prices.

Figure 7.1 **Extent of corruption in four Buenos Aires public hospitals—average of responses by doctors and nurses, 1998 (scale of 0–5)**

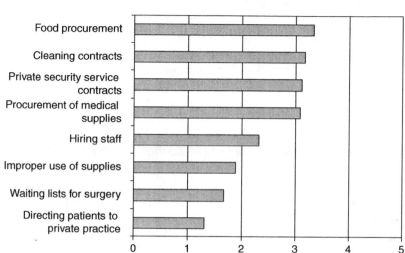

Source: Schargrodsky et al. 2001.
Note: Scores represent the average of responses to the following question: "In your view, what is the level of corruption in public hospitals for the following activities: very high (5), high (4), moderate (3), low (2), very low (1), or non-existent (0)?" [author's translation]. Question was asked to 240 randomly selected doctors and nurses at four hospitals.

A follow-up study distinguished time periods during which the intensity of monitoring varied. That study found that higher wages did reduce corruption in the presence of moderate intensities of auditing. It is reasonable to conclude that the level of pay that purchase managers receive is unlikely to deter them from committing fraud if they face no risk of losing their pay. Impunity undermines any impact that rewards or penalties might have on corruption.

Accountability and Managerial Discretion

In Colombia, hospital supply prices were also used as a proxy for corruption and the findings on purchase managers' income were also inconclusive (Giedion et al. 2001). When this study tested the hypothesis that better-paid managers would be more honest, as indicated by lower purchase prices, it found only a weak negative relationship. Because this weak relationship was an average across different procurement procedures, the researchers separately analyzed prices for supplies that were bid competitively—in which the purchase manager would have more limited discretion to demand bribes—and those that were purchased directly—in which opportunities for corruption are greater. It was expected that higher incomes would have little impact on the procurement that was competitively bid; yet the analysis found that higher-paid managers obtained lower prices with this procedure. It was also expected that higher incomes would be associated with lower prices under direct procurement procedures, yet the analysis found the exact opposite—higher incomes were associated with higher prices paid under direct procurement. Thus, the relationship between purchasing manager's pay and supply prices did not confirm the basic expectation that better pay would be associated with more honest and efficient purchasing.

What the researchers found, instead, was a very strong and consistent impact of two variables that measured accountability: the share of staff with nonpermanent contracts and the share of hospital revenues that came from billing. Hospitals in which fewer staff members have permanent contracts are less constrained when it comes to disciplining workers for infractions, and hospitals that depend on billing for services are constrained in their ability to hide irregularities. Hospital managers, who know their hospital's financial survival depends on revenues that cover expenses, face a strong incentive to limit fraud and abuse when they depend substantially on billing for services. This shows how opportunities to engage in corruption are restricted when individuals and organizations are accountable for their performance.

As in Argentina, low pay might be part of the picture in Bogota's hospitals, but attention to the way the hospitals function, to the incentives they face, and their discretionary authority, tell us a much clearer story. In fact, regardless of staff pay, hospitals with better accountability and greater managerial discretion seem to control corruption better.

And What About Collusion?

In Venezuela, evidence points to an even stranger outcome. Researchers also used unexplained differences in prices for medical supplies as an index of corruption and tested whether higher wages for purchasing managers would be associated with less corruption (Jaén and Paravisini 2001). To their surprise, they found the opposite effect—hospitals that paid their purchase managers more were also the hospitals that paid more for their medical supplies. How is it possible that higher pay would be associated with more corruption?

The study looked for an answer in the probabilities of detection and punishment. It measured the likelihood that corruption would be detected from a survey of hospital staff. Respondents felt that the likelihood of being detected for kickbacks or accepting bribes in procurement was only

31%, compared to 48% for theft and 72% for being absent without an excuse. Beyond these perceptions, the actual experience of impunity was quite widespread—many hospitals reported never having applied sanctions to staff for malfeasance and 40% reported never even investigating the possibility of kickbacks.

As in Argentina, it appears that the absence of effective monitoring and punishment for infractions undercut any potential effect that wages would deter corruption. But in Venezuela, the situation appeared to be even worse. Researchers speculated that the positive association between wages and corruption confirmed widespread suspicion regarding collusion between some hospital directors and purchasing managers. In other words, the normal process in which hospital directors are expected to supervise purchasing managers and ensure that they are acting with integrity had allegedly broken down. Instead, hospital directors were collaborating with corrupt purchasing managers, either indirectly by ignoring evidence of infractions or directly by sharing in the kickbacks or bribes.

Controlling this kind of collusion between supervisors and staff is difficult but not impossible. It requires some form of accountability that is external to the institution. This accountability can be achieved through external performance audits, if a higher-level organization (in this case, the Health Ministry) is ready to investigate and prosecute when malfeasance is found. An independent hospital board can investigate and discipline, or fire, the hospital director on the basis of such evidence. External accountability can also be achieved, however, by a system of incentives that rewards hospitals for performance, a system that was apparently functioning to some extent in Colombia. When hospitals face performance incentives, collusive behavior between management and staff becomes transparent in the form of higher costs and lower productivity.

Low Wages and Absenteeism

Studies of absenteeism among public sector health workers also cast doubt on the claim that higher wages deter corruption. A study of six developing countries in Asia, Africa, and Latin America used a survey with unannounced visits to document the rates of absenteeism (Chaudhury et al. 2006). Not only did they discover high rates of absenteeism but they also found that absenteeism was higher among more highly paid officials. For example, doctors were found to be absent 39% of the time, compared to a rate of 31% for other health workers.

In fact, most studies of absenteeism in the health sector find that higher-paid professionals are more commonly absent than lower-paid staff. Part of this can be explained by the greater opportunities available to highly trained health professionals in terms of seeing private patients. But a large

Figure 7.2 Reported share of hours that staff are absent in Venezuelan hospitals, 1998 (%)

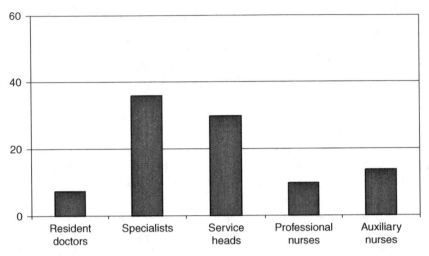

Source: Jaén and Paravisini. 2001.
Note: Responses by doctors and nurses to a survey in 20 Venezuelan hospitals in 1998.

part of the explanation is that higher-paid health professionals are less likely to be punished for their absences. They enjoy higher status in their posts and even play roles in management, supervisory boards, and public sector unions.

In Venezuela, when hospital personnel were surveyed, they reported that specialists were absent about one-third of their contracted hours, whereas head nurses were absent slightly less than 30% of their contracted time (see Figure 7.2). Doctors' absenteeism was partially related to pay in this study but seemed to be particularly responsive to the perceptions of how likely an individual would be detected and punished. It is also of interest that the health professionals with supervisory authority—doctors and head nurses—were reportedly absent three times more often than their subordinates (Jaén and Paravisini 2001).

The significant role of detection and punishment is also found in a study of Colombian hospitals (Giedion et al. 2001). There, absenteeism among doctors was more common in hospitals with a higher share of per-manent staff, that is, staff who had contracts with substantial job security. By contrast, those with time-limited contracts, who could be more easily fired from their jobs, were reportedly absent less often. In the Colombian hospitals, 79% of staff who were surveyed ascribed doctors' absenteeism to either "tolerance of such behavior by the public sector" or "deficient supervisory and control mechanisms," with only 15% blaming low pay (Giedion et al. 2001).

Carrots or Sticks?

It would be a mistake to conclude that wage levels play no role in the likelihood of corruption, but the evidence does show that raising wages in situations of generalized impunity is likely to be ineffective. A first step in any situation might be to assess whether public sector wages are actually low relative to what workers could earn in the private sector. Such evidence can be extremely constructive by clearing debates of fruitless stereotypes (i.e., are civil servants underpaid and hardworking or overpaid and lazy?). Then, based on real information about pay levels, one must examine whether personnel management systems are capable of detecting and punishing malfeasance. A system with impunity is not fair to honest workers or to the people who are entitled to receive public services. Ultimately, when policymakers choose to combat corruption in public services, they are most likely to be successful if they address low pay levels in combination with improving basic audit mechanisms, reducing impunity, and rewarding good performance.

Note

1. This brief draws heavily on research conducted by Ernesto Schargrodsky, Jorge Mera, Federico Weinschelbaum, María Helena Jaén, and Daniel Paravisini as reported in R. Di Tella and W.D. Savedoff, eds. 2001. *Diagnosis corruption: Fraud in Latin America's public hospitals.* Washington, DC: Latin American Research Network, Inter-American Development Bank.

References

Chaudhury, N., J. Hammer, M. Kremer, K. Muralidharan, and F.H. Rogers. 2006. Missing in action: Teacher and health worker absence in developing countries. *Journal of Economic Perspectives* 20, no. 1 (Winter):91–116.

Di Tella, R., and W.D. Savedoff, eds. 2001. *Diagnosis corruption: Fraud in Latin America's public hospitals.* Washington, DC: Latin American Research Network, Inter-American Development Bank.

Ferrinho, P., M.C. Omar, M. de Jesus Fernandez, P. Blaise, A.M. Bugalho, and W. Van Lerberghe. 2004. Pilfering for survival: How health workers use access to drugs as a coping strategy. *Human Resources for Health* 2, no. 4. www.human-resources-health, online access journal.

Filmer, D., and D.L. Lindauer. 2001. Does Indonesia have a low pay civil service? *Bulletin of Indonesian Economic Studies* 37, no. 2:189–205.

Giedion, U., L.G. Morales, and O.L. Acosta. 2001. The impact of health reforms on irregularities in Bogota hospitals. In *Diagnosis corruption: Fraud in Latin America's public hospitals,* ed. R. Di Tella and W.D. Savedoff, chap. 6. Washington, DC: Latin American Research Network, Inter-American Development Bank.

Jaén, M.H., and D. Paravisini. 2001. Wages, capture and penalties in Venezuela's public hospitals. In *Diagnosis corruption: Fraud in Latin America's public hospitals,* ed. R. Di Tella and W.D. Savedoff, chap. 3. Washington, DC: Latin American Research Network, Inter-American Development Bank.

Schargrodsky, E., J. Mera, and F. Weinschelbaum. 2001. Transparency and accountability in Argentina's hospitals. In *Diagnosis corruption: Fraud in Latin America's public hospitals,* ed. R. Di Tella and W.D. Savedoff, chap. 4. Washington, DC: Latin American Research Network, Inter-American Development Bank.

Further Reading

Di Tella, R., and E. Schargrodsky. 2003. The role of wages and auditing during a crackdown on corruption in the city of Buenos Aires. *Journal of Law and Economics* 46, no. 1 (April):269–92.

van Rijckeghem, C., and B. Weder. 2001. Bureaucratic corruption and the rate of temptation: Do wages in the civil service affect corruption, and by how much? *Journal of Development Economics,* 65, no. 2:307–31.

CHAPTER 8

Preventing Drug Diversion Through Supply Chain Management

Taryn Vian

Drug supply is an essential component of health-care systems, accounting for 10–30% of health-care costs. Drugs can be expensive and willingness to pay for drugs is high, creating the danger that employees will take drugs for repackaging and sale in private markets, or for personal use. One carton of an expensive product entering a pharmaceutical warehouse may be worth 5 years' wages for the average warehouse worker and stock loss is a common problem in public sector medical stores, where loss rates often exceed 15%.

The global pandemic of HIV/AIDS, and the commitment to expanding access to antiretroviral treatment in developing countries, creates even greater opportunities for abuse. Antiretroviral drugs are expensive and therefore provide attractive targets for theft and resale. At the same time, mandates to rapidly scale-up treatment programs create pressure to spend funds quickly, increasing the risk of corruption as managers have less time to closely monitor and control drug distribution or update internal controls. Drug supply pipelines that were already weak are now being filled with more product, allowing more opportunity for losses and system breakdown. Oversight is further weakened by the limited supply of health workers (Dräger et al. 2006). As health personnel become sick with AIDS themselves or leave the country in search of a better life, the challenge of finding trained managers and putting in place controls on discretion increases.

Two particular dangers for HIV/AIDS drugs are pharmaceutical arbitrage (also known as parallel trade) and the risk of fake or counterfeit drugs. Although some forms of pharmaceutical arbitrage are legal, in other cases drugs produced and sold at lower prices for distribution by public health-care services are instead illegally diverted and resold for higher profit in the private market. This practice has several negative consequences. First, it reduces the availability of drugs for people who use public facilities, who either forego necessary medications or have to spend large sums to purchase drugs in the private sector. Second, in order to hide this diversion, those who have taken the drugs sometimes replace them with fake or counterfeit drugs. This leads to higher rates of death and morbidity, as well as increasing the development of drug-resistant disease strains. Finally, the sale of diverted drugs in the private market undercuts legitimate sales, undermining the interest of pharmaceutical companies in supplying these markets and limiting availability of essential medicines.

By openly recognizing these risks, public policy can design drug distribution systems to limit the opportunities for such corruption. One such initiative involves the US President's Emergency Plan for AIDS Relief (PEPFAR) and the related Supply Chain Management System (SCMS) project, which are working to increase transparency and provide a secure, high-quality supply of HIV/AIDS drugs to developing countries in Africa and Asia.[1] To achieve this goal, SCMS is promoting commercial best practice in supply chain management. Just as drug manufacturers often contract directly with private distributors to deliver drug orders, the public sectors in Chile, Colombia, Mexico, Peru, and Thailand have contracted with suppliers to deliver drugs directly to service delivery points (WHO Action Programme on Essential Drugs 1998). The management systems used by these private distribution companies are some of the best commercial practices known. This chapter describes some of these practices now being used by Pharmaceutical Healthcare Distributors (PHD) of South Africa, one of the team member organizations in the SCMS project, and similar distributors to provide secure and quality pharmaceutical warehousing and distribution.

Supply Chain Management and PEPFAR

In September 2005, PEPFAR, through the US Agency for International Development, awarded the SCMS contract to strengthen the supply chains providing drugs to treat HIV/AIDS and other infectious diseases in PEPFAR-assisted countries. PEPFAR has purchased over US$350 million in drugs delivered through these supply chains in the first 4 years of the SCMS project. The Partnership for Supply Chain Management Systems is a nonprofit organization established by John Snow Research & Training, Inc. and Management Sciences for Health, Inc. The Partnership has brought together a team of 13 separate organizations from the private sector, academia, and the nonprofit sector to implement SCMS and is well connected to existing delivery and purchasing systems in the developing world.

One of the SCMS team members is PHD of South Africa (www.phdist. co.za). Started in 2000, PHD is a commercial service for drug stockholding and delivery and currently reaches 9,000 delivery points in South Africa on behalf of 30 manufacturers. Services include secure warehousing, inventory management, and drug distribution to individual wholesalers, retailers, hospitals, clinics, and physicians' offices.

Interventions for Transparency in Procurement

SCMS has created a procurement system that follows the US government federal acquisition guidelines. These guidelines promote transparency by requiring public listing of tenders and other procedures so that the procurement is open and competitive.

One key element for transparency in procurement is to make price information publicly available. Having access to the prices paid by drug procurement agencies and distributors is useful to country procurement officers, national audit offices, and international donors as it provides a standard against which to measure other procurements. If a country is procuring drugs at prices that are very different from those published, oversight committees can question why. This creates a deterrent to the bribes and kickbacks that inflate drug prices in many countries.

SCMS has promoted price transparency by establishing an online catalog of prices for items procured under long-term supply contracts negotiated for antiretrovirals and other commonly needed products. Evidence that price transparency works to deter corruption in procurement is available from the hospital price reporting experience in Argentina described in Chapter 9. In that case, the Argentine Ministry of Health tracked prices paid by public hospitals for common drugs, sharing these data with the reporting hospitals. Purchase prices for monitored items immediately fell by an average of 12% (Schargrodsky et al. 2001). Other organizations have implemented strategies for promoting transparency through the publication of comparative price information as well: for example, Management Sciences for Health in collaboration with WHO has been publishing the International Drug Price Indicators Guide since 1986 (Management Sciences for Health and WHO 2005).

Interventions for Secure Distribution

Once drugs have been procured, they must be safely and efficiently delivered through the supply chain to the ultimate consumers. Cost-effective strategies employed successfully by PHD to safeguard drug supply and avoid diversion focus on physical protection and security, segregation of workforce and duties, and risk analysis for dispatch and transportation. In addition, information management can be used to detect diversion of supply from public to private channels. SCMS has adopted some of these best practices in creating a network of regional drug distribution centers for HIV/AIDS commodity distribution located in Ghana, Kenya, and South Africa.

Physical Protection and Security

Physical protection may be the most obvious measure to guard against theft, but it is also frequently neglected or under-funded. Standard measures include locked and gated facilities and compounds, divided areas with controlled access based on drug value, and security guards. When physical security is strong, the most common forms of corruption involve enlisting employees in order to gain access. Sometimes people will specifically seek jobs in pharmaceutical warehouses to be in a position to steal; at other times, employees may be approached and enticed to participate in a corrupt scheme.

Security procedures can guard against these potential risks. First, terms of employment can make clear that all employees will be screened prior to employment, then annually, for credit history and criminal record. In addition, an employer can require that employees take annual polygraphs. Finally, surveillance can protect against the danger that an employee will leave a door unlocked, skip security procedures, sneak out supplies, or otherwise facilitate theft. Overt surveillance may involve guards physically searching employees as they leave the premises and independent checking of orders. Some organizations even use covert monitoring methods, which provide protection by placing paid informant staff in different roles, to listen and report on suspicious activities.

Segregation of Workforce and Duties

In addition to physical protection and security, a distributor can guard against corruption through the segregation of workforce. At PHD, for example, warehouses are divided into three divisions or units, each of which has separate physical areas, personnel policies, and operating procedures. A cage wall separates the Receiving and Warehousing personnel from the Security and Checking staff; another wall separates both these groups of personnel from the Dispatch and Transportation staff. Each division has separate shift times and tea times; personnel wear different colored uniforms, report to different supervisors, and are paid on separate payrolls. Segregating the workforce in this manner prevents collusion and limits discretion.

PHD has applied this principle to the segregation of duties in the order fulfillment, checking, and transport processes as well. Each person has access only to the information they need to fulfill their own tasks. For example, in the Receiving and Warehouse department, the "order picker" (the person who assembles the different products requested by a particular client) knows the product name, bin location, and order quantity but is not aware who the product is for or where it is going. Once the order has been picked, it is moved to Security and Checking unit. Here, the "order checker" (the person who inspects the order for errors and completeness) prints the invoice and places it in the box with the order; the box is then sealed and labeled only with the location. When the box is moved into the Dispatch and Transport department, the dispatch staff and driver only will know where the box is going: they are not given information on the contents or value of the shipment. Cell phones are restricted in the warehouse to prevent sharing information with people outside. When combined, these management procedures create barriers to collusion and corruption.

Dispatch and Transportation

Drugs are also stolen and diverted while in transport. For example, a driver may collude with criminals to drop off some boxes within a shipment or may work with someone to unpack and steal some of the contents of a box. Delivery trucks may also be robbed when traveling high-risk routes, such as routes where robberies have occurred in the past, or where lighting and police presence are scarce.

The risk of theft during transport and delivery is reduced through risk analysis of routes and shipments. Corruption can occur if drivers have been bribed or were planted in the organization (although the danger of this is lessened through the security measures mentioned earlier). On high-risk routes, a distributor may employ higher levels of control and security, with approaches ranging from satellite tracking to interactive driver response or even unmarked escort vehicles to guard delivery trucks. Satellite tracking and monitoring can also provide early warning if a vehicle deviates from the route the driver was scheduled to take. Sophisticated devices can even monitor patterns of braking and acceleration, which can indicate if a delivery truck has been hijacked. Transport dispatchers may phone drivers at regular intervals on very high-risk routes. Finally, some organizations may attach a monitoring device to a high-risk shipment, which allows the shipment to be tracked in the event that it is removed from the transport vehicle prior to the scheduled delivery.

Information Management

Arbitrage, or the diversion of product intended for the public sector to private markets where the pharmaceuticals are sold for a higher price, creates barriers to equitable access to care in addition to reducing margins for pharmaceutical manufacturers. Although it is difficult to measure the extent of the problem, one study in Greece estimated that 22–24% of pharmaceuticals imported or manufactured for consumption in that country were resold into other markets (Kanavos et al. 2004). Applying the lower estimate (22%) to the total pharmaceuticals market in South Africa suggests that up to US$418 million (3.2 billion Rand) may be diverted each year from the public sector to private markets.

Diversion of drug supply can be detected through batch monitoring. Each batch of product that is delivered from a manufacturer to the warehouse is assigned a unique code, which identifies the appropriate channel (i.e., private or public distribution). When products are stocked on shelves and picked for orders, the product that is coded for the public channel will go only to public clients, whereas private channel stock will be packed and shipped to private clients.

Suspected leaks in supply can be investigated by tracing the batch number and checking to make sure that the channel is correct. If the channel is not correct (i.e., if public stock has found its way into private facilities), then further investigation is needed. To trace leaks, it is even possible to deploy covert bar-coded product into a particular distribution channel to obtain evidence.

Packaging technology can be used in combination with investigative activities and legal sanctions to control the problem of diversion of stock. New technology enables a manufacturer, either on its own initiative or to comply with a tender, to print information on the *inside* of the blister pack foil backing used for drug packaging. For some drugs, the message printed on the inside of the foil is "State product, not for sale. If you have paid for this item, it was stolen." Public–private collaboration to deter drug diversion is in the interest of both the government and the manufacturers: government assures increased access to public services by reducing theft of public supplies, whereas the manufacturers assure that products they sell to public procurement agencies at discounted, public sector prices are not being channeled back into private markets. Enforcement activities and community education should be combined with packaging technology interventions, in an integrated approach.

Conclusion

Drugs are expensive and essential to high-quality medical care. With the growing HIV/AIDS pandemic, the market for drugs in the developing world is expanding, creating dangers of drug diversion and the possibility of counterfeit or fake drugs entering public and private markets, especially where government regulatory systems are weak. Poor and vulnerable population groups are most likely to be affected by these problems and to suffer higher morbidity and mortality as a result. Commercial best practice shows that there are logistics management techniques that can safeguard stock. In South Africa, PHD has reduced stock loss to less than 0.1%, providing evidence that investment in preventing diversion can save valuable commodities. These savings can allow more people to be treated. PEPFAR and SCMS are applying commercial best practices to ensure that safe, reliable, high-quality pharmaceutical products get to the patients and consumers who need them, and that supply chains operate in a sustainable manner. In the fight against corruption, it is an effort that deserves our attention and support.

Note

1. This chapter is based on research and interviews with key informants working on drug supply logistics issues. Discussions with Dr. Iain Barton, CEO of Pharmaceutical Healthcare Distributors, Mr. David Jamieson of Crown Agents, and Mr. Richard Owens of SCMS were especially helpful. Mr. Owens reviewed an earlier version of this chapter.

References

Dräger, S., G. Gedik, and M.R. Dal Poz. 2006. Health workforce issues and the Global Fund to fight AIDS, tuberculosis, and malaria: An analytic review. *Human Resources for Health.* 4, no. 23. Open Source journal available online without cost. www.human-resources-health.com/content/4/1/23.

Kanavos, P., J. Costa-i-Font, S. Merkur, and M. Gemmil. 2004. *The economic impact of pharmaceutical parallel trade in European Union member states: A stakeholder analysis.* London: London School of Economics and Political Science. Cited in Lynch K. April 2006. Arbitrage and access: Do measures to stop pharmaceutical arbitrage threaten access to medicines in source countries? Concentration Paper, Department of International Health, Boston, MA.

Management Sciences for Health and WHO. 2005. *International drug price indicator guide.* Boston, MA: Management Sciences for Health. Web-based version available at erc.msh.org/ (accessed September 21, 2009).

Schargrodsky, E., J. Mera, and F. Weinschelbaum. 2001. Transparency and accountability in Argentina's hospitals. In *Diagnosis corruption: Fraud in Latin America's public hospitals,* ed. R. Di Tella and W.D. Savedoff, 116.

Washington, DC: Latin American Research Network, Inter-American Development Bank.

WHO Action Programme on Essential Drugs. 1998. Double issue on managing drug supply. *Essential Drugs Monitor*, nos. 25 and 26: 1–36.

Further Reading

Pharmaceutical Healthcare Distributors (Pty) Ltd. www.phdist.co.za/.

Supply Chain Management Systems (SCMS) Project. www.pfscm.org.

The President's Emergency Plan for AIDS Relief (PEPFAR). www.pepfar .gov/.

CHAPTER 9

The Impact of Information and Accountability on Hospital Procurement Corruption

William D. Savedoff

Hospitals account for a large share of public health expenditures in most countries and procurement of drugs and supplies is one of their larger budget items. Drug procurement alone accounts for 5–10% of hospital expenditures in high-income countries, whereas it can account for as much as 40–60% in low-income settings. It is not surprising, then, to find that within the health sector, hospital procurement is considered highly susceptible to a wide range of scams including kickbacks and delivery of expired and substandard products. In the world's wealthy countries, this may lead to higher costs, but in the world's poorer countries, such corruption can mean the difference between having an equipped facility and one that cannot offer lifesaving treatments.

Studies in different countries show it is possible to investigate and measure this kind of corruption and that publishing information about prices paid for supplies can mitigate the problem. However, the studies also suggest that unless individuals engaging in corrupt practices have some real chance of being detected and punished, information alone is not sufficient to deter corruption.

Buenos Aires Publicizes Hospital Procurement Prices

One of the first steps to detecting problems in hospital procurement is to collect data on prices paid for drugs and supplies. This is exactly what the city government of Buenos Aires did in the late 1990s in order to find out whether procurement was subject to fraud and whether publicizing information about prices would constrain corruption. The experiment has been documented and analyzed in several studies (Di Tella and Schargrodsky 2003; Schargrodsky et al. 2001), showing that many hospitals were overpaying for drugs and supplies and that overpayment declined when price information was disseminated. However, as time passed and no one was investigated or punished for overpayment, purchase prices rose again.

The city government of Buenos Aires operates the second largest hospital network in Argentina. In 1995, it comprised 33 hospitals and 8,375 beds for a population of almost 12 million. At that time, procurement was decentralized to procurement offices in each hospital. Expenditures to maintain and operate these hospitals make up a significant share of the city's budget and when concerns were raised about the possibility of corruption in procurement, the city's Health Secretariat decided to try an experiment. It began to collect information about prices paid for a wide range of nonpharmaceutical medical supplies commonly purchased by hospitals—including needles, syringes, intravenous solutions, x-ray films, and sanitary materials—and announced that it would report this information back to the city's purchasing managers. The first data were collected in August 1996 and the Secretariat began to circulate the price information back to hospital procurement offices in October 1996, allowing them to compare the prices that they paid for supplies with other hospitals. The experiment was eventually stopped in January 1998 when the Secretariat implemented a new accounting system that included new financial controls.

The data revealed very wide dispersion in prices paid for very simple and homogeneous products. For example, the ratio of the highest to lowest prices paid for ethyl alcohol was 10 to 1 (i.e., some hospitals paid prices 10 times higher than what others were paying), whereas for disposable needles, the ratio was 9.5 to 1. Among the 15 products reported by researchers, the lowest ratios were still large—1.8 to 1 for x-ray film (i.e., 80% higher); 2.9 to 1 for physiological solution; and 3.1 to 1 for tubular gas. Even after taking into account differences in volume purchased, terms of payment, and distance between the hospital and the supplier, the prices paid varied widely.

Data collected by the Secretariat showed that the dispersion of prices, as well as the average price, fell quite dramatically in the first months of the experiment (see Figure 9.1). One explanation for the decline in prices could be that corrupt procurement officers feared being discovered, but it could also reflect the response of honest procurement officers who may have been ill informed about the prices available in the market. This latter argument, however, does not explain why the prices fell in September, before the first report on prices was circulated. In other words, prices fell in anticipation that the prices would be reported, not as a consequence of procurement officers learning from the information.

From October 1996 until July 1997, the simple act of collecting and circulating price data appeared to constrain costs and, presumably,

Figure 9.1 Impact of reporting requirements—coefficient of variation for purchase prices in Argentine hospitals

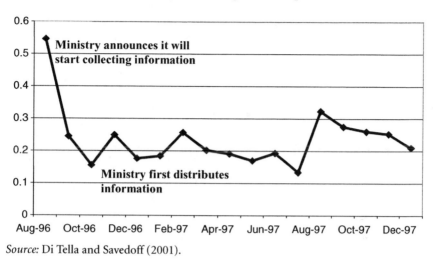

Source: Di Tella and Savedoff (2001).

corruption. Unfortunately, the price range and average increased during the last 5 months of the initiative, suggesting that the impact of information, by itself, was transitory. If the price information were improving efficiency, prices would tend to converge across hospitals. Instead, it seems that procurement officers became accustomed to the process of reporting and began to realize there would be no consequences for "poor performance." In other words, revealing that a particular hospital was overpaying for certain supplies had led to no investigations, reprimands, or additional scrutiny. In the absence of such consequences, it is probable that corrupt individuals resumed their prior illicit activities or that managers became inefficient again. In any case, it did not create incentives for either efficiency or integrity.

Bolivia Promotes Local Accountability

In Bolivia, prices paid by hospitals also varied substantially from one place to the next, but the presence of local hospital boards appears to have constrained corrupt practices involving overpayment for drugs and supplies.

Despite a system of reference prices set by the National Ministry of Health, researchers found that prices paid for homogeneous products varied substantially. For example, in 1998, the Ministry's reference price was US$0.90[1] per liter for sugar water (5% dextrose), but prices paid across

Figure 9.2 Accountability inhibits corruption—range of prices paid for medical supplies in Bolivian hospitals, 1998

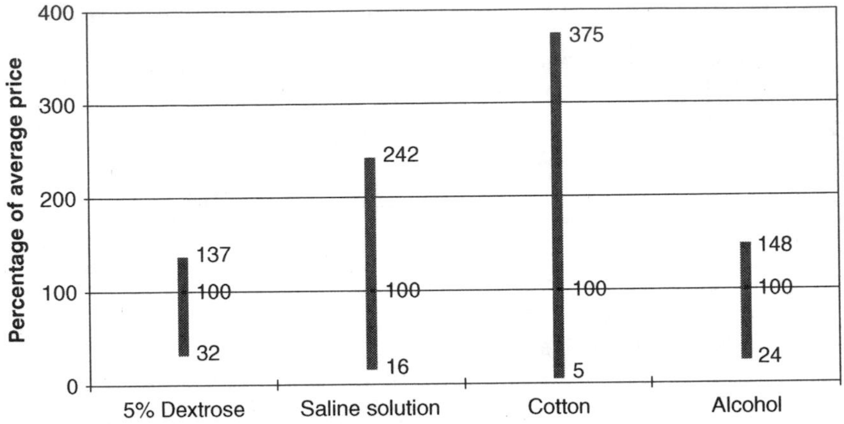

Source: Using data found in Di Tella and Savedoff (2001).

24 municipalities ranged from as low as US$0.36 per liter to as much as US$1.59 per liter (see Figure 9.2). As in Argentina, a study found that the differences in prices could not be explained by differences in volume, terms of payment, or distance to markets (Gray-Molina et al. 2001).

Although Bolivia did not specifically aim to reduce corruption in hospital procurement, another public sector reform in the mid-1990s apparently did have an impact. In that period, Bolivia implemented a national law that devolved numerous responsibilities to municipalities and to representative bodies that included local citizens. Most health-care facilities were handed over to municipalities and supervised by newly created "Local Health Directorates." These directorates included local government officials as well as citizen representatives. Some were quite active, whereas others rarely met or acted.

Researchers collected price data on four different supplies—5% dextrose solution, saline solution, absorbent cotton, and ethyl alcohol—in 30 hospitals and statistically tested whether the presence of active local representatives influenced the hospital's performance in terms of procurement prices. They found that hospitals that were supervised by active directorates paid 40% less on average for 5% dextrose solution. Although paying higher prices is not in itself proof of corruption, the researchers did find that higher prices were correlated with subjective measures of corruption. For example, patients who attended hospitals that paid more for supplies were also likely to view hospitals as more corrupt than other social institutions.

In this case, local supervision appeared to be more effective at controlling corruption than the standard "vertical" controls of the public administration system. Other studies have found the opposite to be true. For example, a study of rural road construction in Indonesia found that increasing the chance of a performance audit significantly reduced corruption in supplying materials, whereas community monitoring had minimal effects (Olken 2005). Efforts to combat corruption, then, have to consider which approach—vertical controls involving hierarchical supervision and audits or horizontal controls involving local community groups and citizens—is likely to be more effective in the particular context.

Rural Doctors Speak Out in Thailand

Thailand's experience shows another case in which horizontal controls effectively confronted corruption; however, in this case, doctors played a key role in mobilizing an entire political campaign to uncover hospital procurement corruption involving very high-level officials. In 1997, Thailand's Minister of Health approved a procedure for centralizing supply procurement and, using the economic crisis that year as an excuse, subsequently suspended a procedural rule aimed at controlling overpayment by hospitals for drugs and medical supplies. Within months, a hospital procurement scandal erupted that eventually forced the minister's resignation (Cameron 2006).

By centralizing procurement, the minister took hospital purchases out of the hands of local health boards that included representatives from the provincial health departments, citizens, and members of the local press. Under the new system, political officeholders had the authority to order provincial staff to purchase drugs and supplies from specific companies. In addition, the elimination of price ceilings made it easier to inflate prices.

Thailand's rural doctors were well organized and responded quickly to concerns over these policy changes. The chairman and former chairman of the Rural Doctors Foundation (RDF), which had been founded in the 1970s, publicized concerns from their members that the new rules were leading to corruption. Along with the Rural Pharmacists Forum (RPF), they conducted surveys to learn what was happening and reported to the press that central officials were forcing provincial officials to purchase drugs and supplies for hospitals at prices two to three times higher than the market price from five specially designated firms. When the government did not respond, RDF mobilized a political campaign involving a coalition of 30 NGOs. Using the press and the courts, this coalition was able to obtain incriminating information and force the creation of an independent investigative committee. The investigation led two ministers to resign and to the dismissal of several senior and mid-level officials.

This experience shows, first, that hospital procurement can be corrupted by individuals outside as well as within the hospital. It shows how collecting information and publicizing it can bring corruption to the public attention and, perhaps most significantly, it shows how important it is for societies to have organized civil society groups with sufficient legitimacy to confront the government when corruption is discovered. Thailand had all these ingredients and the effort to corrupt hospital procurement was thwarted.

Conclusions

The stories of corruption in hospital procurement are not exclusive to Argentina, Bolivia, and Thailand but occur throughout the world (Vian 2006). The most common thread in most cases is that corruption is common wherever impunity is the rule.

The Argentine case demonstrates that shining light in dark corners can modify behaviors initially, but unless publicizing information has some consequences—whether through convictions, loss of employment, disciplinary actions, or moral disapprobation—the gains from publicizing corruption may be short lived. The Bolivian case suggests that active local oversight can modify behaviors as well, though the study did not follow the cases to see if these gains were sustained. Thailand's experience shows the feasibility of gathering information from health-care workers when professional associations are organized to monitor and question governmental authorities. All three cases show that collecting data provides hard facts that can reveal corruption. To reduce corruption, though, requires accountability—action in response to those facts.

Note

1. In 1998, the exchange rate was approximately 5.5 bolivianos per US dollar.

References

Cameron, S. 2006. Corruption in the Ministry of Public Health, Thailand. In *Global corruption report 2006: Special focus: Corruption and health*, ed. Transparency International, 100–1. London and Ann Arbor, MI: Pluto Press.

Di Tella, R., and E. Schargrodsky. 2003. The role of wages and auditing during a crackdown on corruption in the city of Buenos Aires. *Journal of Law and Economics*, 46, no. 1 (April): 269–92.

Gray-Molina, G., E. Pérez-Rada, and E. Yañez. 2001. Does voice matter? Participation and controlling corruption in Bolivian hospitals. In *Diagnosis corruption: Fraud in Latin America's public hospitals*, ed. R. Di Tella and W.D. Savedoff, 27–55. Washington, DC: Latin American Research Network, Inter-American Development Bank.

Olken, B.A. 2007. Monitoring corruption: Evidence from a field experiment in Indonesia. *Journal of Political Economy* 115, no. 2 (April): 200–49.

Schargrodsky, E., J. Mera, and F. Weinschelbaum. 2001. Transparency and accountability in Argentina's hospitals. In *Diagnosis corruption: Fraud in Latin America's public hospitals*, ed. R. Di Tella and W.D. Savedoff, 95–122. Washington, DC: Latin American Research Network, Inter-American Development Bank.

Vian, T. 2006. Corruption in hospitals. In *Global corruption report 2006: Special focus: Corruption and health*, ed. Transparency International, 49–61. London and Ann Arbor, MI: Pluto Press.

CHAPTER 10

Transparency and Accountability in an Electronic Era: The Case of Pharmaceutical Procurement

Brenda Waning and Taryn Vian

Since 2002, development assistance for health has grown dramatically, driven in part by the HIV/AIDS pandemic and the growth of global health initiatives such as the US President's Emergency Plan for AIDS Relief (PEPFAR), the Global Fund to Fight AIDS, Tuberculosis, and Malaria (the Global Fund), and the Global Alliance for Vaccines and Immunization (GAVI) (Ravishankar et al. 2009). The expansion in funding for global health means that more labor and financial resources are being dedicated to the procurement of medicines for treatment. While patients, physicians, national governments, and development partners are eager to see treatment programs expanded, rapid scale-up often results in circumstances whereby resources have to be spent quickly, and sometimes resources are added to systems that are already weak and vulnerable to corruption. Program expansion in these circumstances can result in more risk, waste, and losses, especially in the procurement process. Price transparency is the first step toward identifying and minimizing corruption in procurement. This chapter describes how international partners and national procurement agencies have used information technology to improve transparency and increase accountability in procurement of HIV/AIDS medicines.

Background

After personnel, pharmaceuticals are the largest category of health expenditure in many countries. It is no surprise, then, that procurement of medicines is vulnerable to inefficiencies and corruption. Problems are due to many factors, including untrained staff, inability to draft proper bidding documents, delayed payments to suppliers, and national procurement laws that are not specifically designed to handle pharmaceuticals. Inefficiencies in procurement can also be a result of corruption. Bribes and other corrupt practices can influence the choice of seller, the quantities of medicines procured, the prices paid, and the quality of medicines purchased. In rich and poor countries alike, the ability to detect and address these issues is hampered by a lack of transparency in medicine prices. Historically, the pharmaceutical industry has intentionally not published information on medicine prices, making it difficult for purchasers to negotiate a fair price. The secrecy that shrouds medicine prices also makes it difficult to hold procurement staff accountable for good procurement practices. This information asymmetry, combined with procurement systems that allow critical decisions to be made by a few powerful people, creates environments prone to corruption.

Recent advances in information technology have kindled interest in improving transparency in drug price information. For example, it is becoming increasingly common for countries and donors to manage and store drug procurement information in electronic format. These drug procurement databases have great potential to advance the transparency agenda in pharmaceuticals. Yet transparency is achieved only if data are consistently reported, reliable in terms of quality, and in a format that can be used to identify potential issues. Furthermore, transparency is effective only to the extent that agents are held accountable when they overpay for drugs. In this chapter we describe how Boston University (BU) researchers drew on publicly available data from the Global Fund and the World Health Organization (WHO) Global Price Reporting Mechanism (GPRM) to improve transparency in medicines procurement by strengthening data quality, creating performance indicators and benchmarking reports, and promoting public dialogue.

Advances in Transparency of Medicine Procurements

While most major donors require that procurements be reported in order to receive funding, no other donors disclose antiretroviral (ARV) procurement information with as much transparency as the Global Fund. The unprecedented policies and procedures implemented by the Global Fund have changed the landscape around transparency of medicine procurements. All medicine and commodity procurements made through Global Fund programs must be reported by the principal recipients and then posted on the Global Fund's publicly available website.[1]

Some procurements not reported through the Global Fund's system are nonetheless available through another public database, the GPRM managed by the WHO.[2] The GPRM contains procurements reported by non-Global Fund programs such as PEPFAR, as well as procurements reported by international procurement agencies and the Global Fund. Because the GPRM includes the Global Fund and non-Global Fund programs, it now serves as a global data repository on medicine procurements for HIV/AIDS, tuberculosis, and malaria.

Transparency and Accountability

Information on medicines procurement is useful for many purposes, including planning, policy setting, management decision making, and transparency. However, to improve public deliberation and accountability, disclosure of information by web posting is not enough. A fully operational policy on transparency also requires that information be consistently reported and consistently accessible, of reliable quality, standardized, comparable, and disaggregated to further a defined public purpose (Brinkerhoff 2004). Clear, easy-to-understand, and timely information must be provided to people who can use it to hold public or private institutions accountable.

While the Global Fund and WHO have vastly improved transparency of ARV procurements by making transactions publicly available on the web, these data have not been extensively used. A survey conducted by WHO reported that more than 50% of the intended audience for the database rarely or never accesses it (Samb 2007). Underuse of these data is likely to be related to a combination of factors, including a lack of awareness that such data exist in the public domain, a lack of knowledge in how such information can be used, and issues around data quality and user-friendliness.

How can the public health community move from mere transparency toward external accountability in how procurements of ARV medicines unfold? To address this question, we need to consider the three key elements of transparency: the discloser, the information being disclosed, and the recipient of the information. Intervening in each of these elements can make transparency more effective and improve accountability.

Increasing Coverage of Who Discloses

Optimal use of these data for promoting transparency will require higher levels of reporting compliance among Global Fund recipients (currently estimated to be only 30–35%) and a mandate from other donors that procurements be reported to WHO GRPM. This expands the number of organizations disclosing and the scope of procurements disclosed.

Improving the Reliability and Accuracy of Data

Multiple spellings, misspellings, confusion around definitions of data labels, and data entry errors need to be eliminated at the point of data entry.

Design features such as drop-down menu options, which minimize the use of free text data entry, should be incorporated, and forms pilot tested to ensure consistent interpretation of items.

Data verification routines should be built into systems to minimize erroneous data entries for variables such as price, which do not lend themselves to drop-down menus. Automated price verification would signal a warning message when prices reported are far in excess of prices in the database for the identical product, and ask for verification before accepting the report.

Assuring Consistent, Reliable Access to Disclosed Information in a Practical Format

Access to web-based data must be consistent and reliable. Considerations should be made to avoid system downtime and to address the limited Internet connectivity that exists for users in low-resource settings. In addition, indicators need to be created, which transform raw data into performance measures, and which communicate how particular procurements or countries stack up against standards or against the performance of others.

Moving Forward on the Transparency Agenda

Researchers at Boston University, with funding from the United Kingdom's Department for International Development, have been helping implement some of these recommendations for moving from transparency to accountability, building on the work of WHO and the Global Fund. First, the Global Fund database and the WHO GPRM database were merged into a single data set to ensure all reported ARV procurements were captured. Next, the merged data set was extensively cleaned to remove erroneous and duplicate entries. New variables were added to allow for more robust analysis. Overall, the improved database contained more than 5,000 procurement transactions for the time period November 2002 through June 2006, totaling over US$230 million. The data include 27 variables providing detailed ARV procurement information on country, region, products, manufacturers, suppliers, mode of delivery, product quality, price, and participation in price-negotiation and differential pricing schemes.

In addition to cleaning and expanding the data, researchers developed tools to measure and assess relative efficiency within and between countries around ARV procurement. These differences in efficiency could be a result of mismanagement and, possibly, of intentional corruption. As the "essence of accountability is answerability," funding organizations and supervisors should use these indicators to ask questions, and procurement officers should be able to explain variation in prices or gaps in efficiency. Through this process, it is possible to identify when individuals may require further training and professional development, when system-wide reforms are necessary, and when criminal investigations should be started.

The two main transparency tools that BU helped to create are high price outlier analysis and country benchmarking of prices paid.

High Price Outlier Analysis

The first transparency tool, high price outlier analysis, conducted on each ARV, allows information users to quickly zero in on procurements whose prices are far in excess of the global distribution of prices paid for that same product. In the BU study, researchers identified 80 high price outliers over the time period November 2002–June 2006.

High price outlier reports can be used internally by donor programs to screen procurements and identify potential problems. Once a potential problem is identified, further investigation can determine the factors that contributed to the excessively high prices. Examples of high price outlier analyses are provided pictorially as histograms in Figures 10.1 and 10.2, where price per tablet is plotted on the x axis and the number of procurements for that product is plotted on the y axis. In Figure 10.1, the bulk of procurements for lamivudine 150 mg are clustered on the left side of the

Figure 10.1 High price outlier analysis, Lamivudine 150 mg

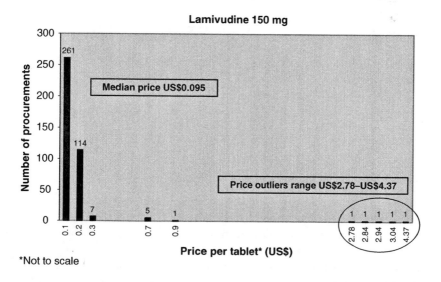

*Not to scale

Figure 10.2 High price outlier analysis, Nevirapine 200 mg

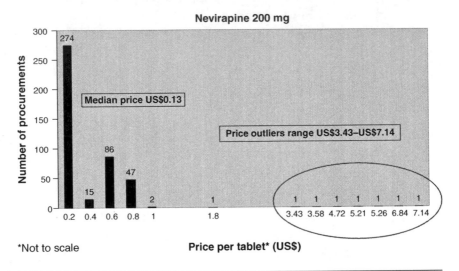

*Not to scale

graph, with most prices paid ranging between US$0.05 and US$0.33 per tablet. But on the far right side of the chart are scattered procurements where countries paid US$2.94, US$3.04, and US$4.37 for the same product. These severe price variations are not easily explained as natural price variations in the market.

Figure 10.2 is perhaps the most striking example of price outlier analysis. In this histogram, the price distribution for nevirapine 200 mg shows a bimodal distribution, with generic prices ranging from US$0.07 to US$0.40 and brand prices ranging from US$0.63 to US$0.75, but in the far right are price outliers where prices paid ranged from US$3.43 to US$7.14 per tablet. In this example, one may investigate not only why a country would pay high outlier prices but also why a country would choose to purchase a brand name product that is considerably more expensive than equivalent generic products.

Country Benchmarking of Prices Paid for ARVs

The second transparency tool that can be used to assess prices paid for medicines is a benchmark that compares prices paid in-country to global median prices paid for identical products. The BU researchers benchmarked all 90 countries in the database but for clarity report only a sample of 8 countries here (with names removed to focus attention on the tool). In Table 10.1, the percentages of country procurements are

**Table 10.1 Global price distribution country performance,
July 2005–June 2006**

COUNTRY (WHO REGION)	% OF COUNTRY PROCUREMENTS ACROSS QUARTILES OF GLOBAL PRICE DISTRIBUTION			
	4TH (HIGHEST) QUARTILE	3RD QUARTILE	2ND QUARTILE	1ST (LOWEST) QUARTILE
Countries with lowest performance				
Country A (E. Europe)	100			
Country B (S. America)	80	20		
Country C (C. Asia)	82		9	9
Country D (Sub-Saharan Africa)	58	8	17	17
Countries with highest performance				
Country E (W. Africa)		25	17	58
Country F (W. Africa)		4	32	64
Country G (Caribbean)	4	12	44	40
Country H (E. Europe)	21	3	14	62

described across quartiles of the global price distribution for the time period July 2005–June 2006. The quartiles are defined by dividing the sorted prices into four parts, each representing one-fourth of the sample. Thus, the lowest quartile includes the lowest 25% of prices paid, the second quartile includes prices that were in the 26–50% percentile, the third quartile includes prices in the 51–75% percentile, and the highest quartile contains prices above the 75th percentile. In this distribution, it is desirable for countries to have the majority of their procurements ranked in the lowest or second quartile, meaning their prices were at or below global median prices for identical products. Countries would prefer to avoid rankings in the third or highest quartiles, meaning the prices they paid were above global median prices for identical products.

In this example, all of country A's procurements were priced in the highest quartile, the most expensive category. Further investigation is necessary to determine whether this country is consistently paying higher prices for all its ARV procurements for legitimate reasons (e.g., transportation costs are high), for reasons related to poor management (e.g., bids are not reviewed properly), or as a result of kickbacks, bid-rigging, bribes, or other fraud. By contrast, the bottom half of Table 10.1 shows the four countries with the highest number of procurements priced in the lowest quartile of all global prices for identical products. More than 60% of procurements in countries F and H were priced in the lowest quartile. Further investigation of these cases might reveal best practices in pharmaceutical procurement that could be emulated elsewhere, though one should be careful to assure that the drugs being procured are of good quality. Low prices may also indicate that companies have skimped on active agents or relabeled expired drugs (Akunyili 2006).

Conclusion

Conventional wisdom suggests improvements in transparency will lead to improved efficiency and decreased opportunities for corruption in pharmaceutical procurement. Yet transparency is only a first step on the road to accountability. Information systems create opportunities to advance the transparency agenda through public disclosure of procurement information via the World Wide Web, but high-level political commitment is needed to mandate, enforce, and disclose procurement reports. Procurement information must be accurate, consistently accessible, and user-friendly. More work is needed to transform valuable raw procurement data into information tools to facilitate and monitor procurement at program, country, and donor levels. This case brief provides illustrative examples of the types of tools that could be developed using existing data sources. Once the appropriate tools have been developed, they need to be incorporated into monitoring and evaluation systems that enable excessive prices to be identified and further investigated. Linking transparency to accountability in this way can help curb corruption and further goals of expanded access to essential medicines.

Notes

1. Global Fund to Fight AIDS, TB, and Malaria. www.theglobalfund. org/en/ (accessed August 25, 2009).

2. World Health Organization Global Price Reporting Mechanism. www.who.int/hiv/amds/gprm/en/ (accessed August 25, 2009).

References

Akunyili, D. 2006. The fight against counterfeit drugs in Nigeria. In *Global corruption report 2006: Special focus: Corruption and health*, ed. Transparency International, chap. 5, 96–100. London and Ann Arbor, MI: Pluto Press.

Brinkerhoff, D. 2004. Accountability and health systems: Toward conceptual clarity and policy relevance. *Health Policy and Planning* 19, no. 6: 371–9.

Ravishankar, N., P. Gubbins, R.J. Cooley, K. Leach-Kemon, C.M. Michaud, D.T. Jamison and C.J. Murray. 2009. Financing of global health:

Tracking development assistance for health from 1990 to 2007. *The Lancet* 373, no. 9681:2113–24.

Samb, B. 2007. The bottlenecks towards uninterrupted access to medicines and diagnostics. Presentation to WHO technical consultation meeting on the relevance and modalities of implementation of an observatory for HIV commodities in Africa, Durban, South Africa, June 2007.

Further Reading

Eaton, L. 2005. Global Fund toughens stance against corruption. *British Medical Journal* 331:718.

WHO Good Governance for Medicines Programme website and publications. www.who.int/medicines/ggm/en/ (accessed September 16, 2009).

PART FOUR

Restoring Integrity Through Transparency and Accountability

CHAPTER 11

Transparency in Health Programs

Taryn Vian

Transparency is an important tool for good governance, helping to expose abusive practices including fraud, patronage corruption, and other abuses of power. Increasing transparency can also enhance accountability by providing performance information and exposing policies and procedures to oversight. This chapter discusses the role of transparency in preventing corruption in the health sector.

Transparency and Good Governance

Board members and management teams in public and private health organizations occupy positions of trust and are responsible for exercising entrusted power in pursuit of collective interests. Whether the groups whose interests they represent are citizens or shareholders, employees or donors, the governance structures of these organizations require that officials do not abuse their power or positions for personal gain. One way to ensure that such officials do not abuse their positions is to make information about their activities available to those who can hold them accountable. In this way, transparency not only limits abuses, it also encourages communication that is necessary for improving organizational decisions and performance, and it provides a lever for increasing stakeholder engagement. Yet, transparency is not always easy to implement. Who is really responsible for transparency? What information should be shared, and with whom? To answer these questions, we must first examine the definition of transparency and its different components.

What Is Transparency?

According to Transparency International, transparency is "a principle that allows those affected by administrative decisions, business transactions,

105

or charitable work to know not only the basic facts and figures but also the mechanisms and processes. It is the duty of civil servants, managers, and trustees to act visibly, predictably, and understandably" (Transparency International 2009).

By this definition, transparency is a code of conduct or a set of rules to guide actions by responsible officials. Looking closely at this definition, we see that transparency involves four things: something disclosed or communicated, an observer or recipient of the disclosed information, a discloser or person whose actions are being observed, and a means for the disclosure to take place.

Disclosure of Information

The first element of a transparency code involves the *disclosure of information*, either proactively or when requested by someone who has a right to know. Freedom of information (also called access to information) legislation obliges governments to make information publicly available, including information about budgets and organizational practices, unless there is a compelling reason to restrict it (e.g., national security). When governments conceal or withhold information, freedom of information laws generally establish procedures under which citizens or civil society organizations can request information based on their legal rights of access. In countries with appropriate checks and balances, this can function well. For example, the newspaper *La Nación* in Costa Rica requested information about the noncontributory pensions accorded to board members of a social service agency. Although the government initially denied the request, the court agreed that the journalists did have a constitutional right to this information and compelled the government to disclose it (Transparency International 2006, 148). Croatia, Ecuador, Guatemala, and Serbia all have recognized the right of citizens to access public information, although in each country more work is needed to assure that legitimate requests are fulfilled in a timely way.

In recent years, more health organizations—both public and private— are adopting *active disclosure* policies, imposing transparency on themselves as a way to prove they are trustworthy, increase performance, and reduce risk of corruption (Fung et al. 2007). Active disclosure policies do not require citizens to make requests. A study of budget transparency in 36 countries found that although virtually all countries make the executive's budget proposal publicly available, 25% did not make routine budget monitoring reports available, and 33% did not release audit reports (Transparency International 2006, 316–7). Yet, this information is essential in order to hold governments accountable for budget performance and to have informed debate about fiscal priorities.

For full transparency, the information disclosed should include not only the "facts and figures" but also the "mechanisms and processes" by which the work is accomplished. Understanding how decisions were made may be just as important as what was decided or done when evaluating the performance of someone in a position of authority. Applying this principle to an immunization program, we might ask not only how many children were immunized, but also why mobile clinics were held in some villages but not in others. In addition to reporting how much was spent on immunization, the government should explain how it determined the quantities of vaccines to purchase, or how it chose the suppliers used. Table 11.1 gives an example of information that can be disclosed to promote transparency in the areas of budgets, medicines, and human resources.

Observer's Right to Know

The second aspect of a transparency code is identifying the observer or recipient. Access to information is to be granted to those *affected* by the decisions, transactions, or work. In the health sector, this could include a range of stakeholders, including health center employees, patients, donors or funding agencies, other government offices, and citizen advocacy groups. Organizations that follow the active disclosure model of transparency should give thought to which audiences are affected by their actions and try to target release of data specifically to these audiences.

A Duty to Disclose?

A third aspect of a transparency code defines the *disclosers* of information. These are the civil servants (government agents), managers, and trustees who hold positions of responsibility and make decisions on behalf of shareholders, taxpayers, beneficiaries, or citizens. By declaring that disclosers have a "duty" to act visibly, predictably, and understandably vis à vis the stakeholders or information recipients, a transparency code implies that the disclosers are in a position of trust and have obligations toward the stakeholders or the recipients of information.

In the health sector, the idea that such obligations to others establish a responsibility to be transparent also extends to doctors, nurses, pharmacists, and other clinical workers, whether or not they work in the public sector. However, a difficult balance must sometimes be struck between the goal of transparent conduct and the need to protect the privacy of patients. Procedures to remove patient-identifying information or pool data are often necessary to assure that confidentiality is not breached.

Acting *visibly* suggests that the civil servants, managers, and trustees should not be hiding anything that is part of their institutional or fiduciary

Table 11.1 Information for transparency

AREA FOR TRANSPARENCY	FACTS AND FIGURES	MECHANISMS AND PROCESSES
Budgets	• Budget requested, amount approved, and funds received • Share of budgeted amount received within 1 month of budget approval	• What is the timing of the budget process? • How are priorities set for which programs or geographic regions will receive funding? • What are causes for delays?
Medicines	• Quantity procured • Unit prices paid • Suppliers used • Share of procurements at or below the average international procurement price	• What kind of bidding process is used? • Who is involved in the selection of the winning supplier? • How does the organization decide how much to order?
Human resources	• Number and names of personnel of each level • Job descriptions and qualifications for staff • Share of staff who are qualified for post	• How are job openings circulated? • How are job finalists selected? • What are the criteria used to determine satisfactory or unsatisfactory performance, or to award promotions?
Quality of care and patient satisfaction	• Top five problems cited by patients • Share of patients who reported being forced to make an informal payment in order to receive care	• What aspects of the patient care process are responsible for the problems cited? • How are patient complaints recorded and handled?

role (though they may still claim a right to privacy with respect to their personal lives). For these same people to act *predictably* means that others can see the probable impact of the officials' actions before the actions are taken. Finally, acting *understandably* implies that the people affected by the actions can account for the *motivations* and *interests* of the person in the position of trust (the civil servant, manager, or trustee) and can assess or judge how the motivations and interests led to the actions.

Means of Disclosure

The fourth aspect of a transparency code is the means of disclosure. As organizations consider ways to improve transparency, they must decide what format the disclosure should take, and the methods to be used in communicating or sharing information. Format includes whether the information is raw data (which allows for multiple analyses by the consumer), processed indicators, or analytical and interpretive reports. Whenever possible, it is best to provide all three of these because they will be useful to different audiences. Having access to the underlying data makes it possible for individuals or organizations to test whether interpretations in reports are supported by the raw data. In addition to performance indicator data, policy documents, procedure manuals, and minutes of meetings are data formats that help illuminate the "mechanisms and processes" by which decisions are made.

Dissemination channels can include face-to-face meetings, such as staff meetings, board meetings, or advisory committee meetings. Information can also be transmitted via websites, e-mail listservs, newspaper notices, and documents made available in public places (e.g., posted in health facilities) or by mail.

Examples of Transparency in the Health Sector

The health sector is complex and involves a wide range of public and private actors. One article specifically identified 11 different parties who can be held accountable or hold others accountable in the health sector, including physicians, government, private payers, employers, investors, managed care plans, hospitals, professional associations, lawyers and courts, and patients (Emanuel and Emanuel 1996). For this reason, transparency in the sector involves many kinds of information collected and disseminated by and to different individuals and organizations. Some examples of ways in which transparency has been used to enhance accountability include controlling the influence of pharmaceutical companies on physicians through transparency on gift-giving practices; promoting better hospital care through citizen report cards; reducing misappropriation of public resources through transportation logs; and improving performance of mandatory health insurers.

In the United States, professional associations of the pharmaceutical industry and physicians have set limits on gift-giving to protect medical decisions from being unduly biased. To monitor compliance with these codes of conduct, some state governments have passed laws mandating disclosure of payments to doctors by pharmaceutical companies. The disclosure laws promote transparency by assuring that the motivations and interests of the doctors and pharmaceutical companies are open to public scrutiny. However, when a university research team tried to access the information collected by government, they encountered many problems (Ross et al. 2007). In Vermont, data were available in summarized form but not by individual doctor. The researchers had to submit a request under the Freedom of Information Act to access the full data set and experienced a long delay. In addition, pharmaceutical companies were allowed to designate some payments as "trade secrets" that the government could use internally but not disclose to the public. In Minnesota, the researchers were able to obtain copies of the actual forms filled in by pharmaceutical companies, but data had never been entered into a computer or analyzed by the state, and forms were incomplete or contained errors. The researchers made several recommendations for how to achieve the intended effect of the disclosure law. Recommendations included disallowing the "trade secret exemption," assigning one state agency to be responsible for collecting, analyzing, and reporting the disclosed information, providing penalties for noncompliance, and requiring the state to make data available to the public in an "understandable" manner (Ross et al. 2007).

Since the research was published, several policy changes were made. In Minnesota, the disclosures are now available in pdf format through the Internet, an initial step toward the goal of having a web-searchable system. In Vermont, the trade secret designation was struck down, allowing all disclosures to become public. The government has also improved consistency in reporting the names of doctors who received payments and is collecting additional data on the medication for which the payment was made. The publicity surrounding this study has played a role in the development of the Physician Payment Sunshine Act, a proposed law (S.103, 111th Congress, 1st Session 2009), which combines many of the elements of the Minnesota and Vermont programs, and which has been introduced in the US Senate as part of national health reform initiatives (Physician Payments Sunshine Act of 2009).

Creating "report cards" for hospitals and health facilities is another mechanism to promote transparency, in this case for the purpose of encouraging better quality care. Report cards are sometimes created by consumer watchdog agencies, private companies, insurance agencies, or government offices. Examples include the Colorado Hospital Report Card (www.cohospitalquality.org), whose stated purpose is to make hospital quality data available to the general public "in a clear and usable manner," and the Bangalore Citizen Report Cards, implemented by the nonprofit Public Affairs Centre (PAC) of Bangalore, India. In 2000, PAC created a report card to measure health-care services serving the urban poor. The report card indicated low patient satisfaction, poorly maintained facilities, and widespread corruption in the form of bribes and under-the-table payments for care. The study reported that only 43% of patients had access to usable toilets, and less than 40% had access to free medicines as required by government policy. PAC used this information to put pressure on the municipality. It then worked with the Bangalore Municipal Corporation to implement reforms. An evaluation in 2004 found that services had significantly improved: cleaning and laundry functions had been outsourced for better accountability, qualified nurses had replaced untrained staff, a board of overseers had been created with elected councilors and prominent citizen members, and a citizen charter was in place, defining rights of patients (Ravindra 2004). A Citizen Report Card Project in Uganda similarly found that a transparency initiative increased quality and quantity of health-care service provision and improved health outcomes such as increased immunization rates and reduced waiting time (Gauthier and Reinikka 2007, 43–4).

Transparency can promote better performance and combat waste and fraud when it is used to increase the visibility of staff performance within an organization. For example, in Ghana, the Ministry of Health was concerned with possible misuse of vehicles and fuel supplies. Ministry officials asked transport officers to calculate fuel utilization and display the results on a notice board. Immediately after the information was posted, average fleet fuel utilization jumped from 5.5 to 6.3 km/L, a 15% improvement. As this initiative continued over several years, a 70% improvement in fuel utilization was eventually achieved, dramatically reducing vehicle running costs. In contrast, researchers noted that in Cote d'Ivoire, lack of vehicle logbooks concealed abuses such as fuel fraud and unauthorized use of vehicles, making it difficult to hold managers accountable (Abt Associates 2001, 27).

Transparency also plays an important role in the governance of mandatory health insurance systems in Estonia and Chile (Savedoff and Gottret 2008). Both countries established requirements for regular reporting of financial data and performance figures to their boards and to financial authorities, while Estonia established a balanced scorecard linking the use of resources to the achievement of performance goals. In addition, both countries have used the Internet to make financial and performance data available for public oversight.

Other examples show the broad range of transparency initiatives, which can improve accountability in use of public resources. According to WHO, sharing "white lists" of reliable and prequalified suppliers and sharing information on prices paid puts downward pressure on prices bid by suppliers and helps to reduce opportunities for bribes. Making hospital waiting lists public is a strategy being used in Croatia, to reduce the practice of patients bribing doctors to jump ahead in the queue. Analysis of publicly available budget information in Nigeria helped to debunk officials' claims that staff nonpayment was due to budget allocations being insufficient, demonstrating instead that funds had been diverted unjustifiably.

Challenges

Although the advantages to transparency are clear, transparency initiatives also have costs and challenges for sustainability. Programs to facilitate regular releases of high-quality, understandable information, and to make it available easily to those affected by decisions, can be expensive: for example, each Bangalore report card took 7 months and cost up to US$12,000 to produce. As described in Chapter 10, it took over 6 months to produce a usable comparative database of HIV/AIDS medicines procurement data, and further training and systems improvement continue to be needed to achieve full transparency in drug pricing information.

Transparency initiatives should be designed to minimize recurrent costs by focusing on the release of already collected government data, including budget documents, audit reports, and utilization data. In addition, report cards or other efforts in active disclosure should use standardized systems for data collection, reporting, and information dissemination, which build on regular government operations. More work is needed to assess the costs of alternative interventions to achieve transparency and to quantify the cost savings from fraud and abuse prevented.

Conclusion

Transparency is an essential feature of good governance and a means for preventing abuse of power in the health sector. Achieving the goal of greater transparency in health-care organizations requires that concerned stakeholders first develop a common understanding of transparency, before settling on priorities and strategies for implementation. By defining the information to be disclosed, the observer, the discloser, and the means for communicating information, organizations can achieve consensus on what transparency means and how to implement it effectively.

References

Abt Associates, Inc., Bill and Melinda Gates Children's Vaccine Program, WHO. February 2001. Transport in Primary Healthcare, Composite Report.

Emanuel, E.J., and L.L. Emanuel. 1996. What is accountability in health care? *Annals of Internal Medicine* 124, no. 2:229–39.

Fung, A., M. Graham, and D. Weil. 2007. *Full disclosure: The perils and promise of transparency.* New York: Cambridge University Press.

Gauthier, B., and R. Reinikka. 2007. Methodological approaches to the study of institutions and service delivery: A review of PETS, QSDS and CRCS. African Economic Research Consortium Framework paper. August.

Physician Payments Sunshine Act of 2009, S.301, 11th Congress, 1st Session, 2009.

Ravindra, A. 2004. An assessment of the impact of Bangalore Citizen Report Cards on the performance of public agencies. ECD Working Paper Series 12, World Bank, Washington, DC.

Ross, J.S., J.E. Lackner, P. Lurie, C.P. Gross, S. Wolfe, and H.M. Krumholz. 2007. Pharmaceutical company payments to physicians: Early experiences with disclosure laws in Vermont and Minnesota. *JAMA.* 297, no. 11:1216–23.

Savedoff, W.D., and P. Gottret. 2008. *Governing mandatory health insurance: Learning from experience.* Washington, DC: World Bank.

Transparency International. 2006. *Global corruption report 2006: Special focus: Corruption and health.* London and Ann Arbor, MI: Pluto Press.

Transparency International. 2009. www.transparency.org/news_room/faq/corruption_faq (accessed August 25, 2009).

CHAPTER 12

Using Financial Performance Monitoring to Promote Transparency and Accountability in Health Systems

David Collins and Taryn Vian

Health sector corruption is difficult to uncover because it takes so many forms and because those involved try to hide their tracks. As discussed in other chapters, internal controls and audits are an important way to strengthen financial systems so that corruption can be detected and prevented. However, standard financial monitoring is limited in what it can find. Fortunately, systems that measure and report on the linkages between financial flows and service delivery, that is, "financial performance monitoring," can uncover a wide range of problems. Once such systems are functioning, they increase transparency in ways that deter abuse.

This chapter discusses financial performance monitoring and how it can help deter health sector corruption. Drawing on the experiences of district health management teams in South Africa, the chapter discusses interventions to improve district health planning and reporting systems, including the integration of financial data and service utilization statistics and the use of standard cost comparisons. We describe how these strategies enhanced transparency and accountability and focused managerial attention on areas vulnerable to abuse.

Financial Monitoring Systems: Challenges and Options

Monitoring financial performance is part of an overall set of management control systems. Improved monitoring can help to increase the probability that anomalies will be identified and can help quantify the magnitude of the problem. Stronger management control and reporting can help curb not just corruption, but inefficiency as well, providing incentives for more rigorous and accountable management.

Despite these potential benefits, financial monitoring in many developing countries today is limited to comparing actual expenditures with budgets. This rarely detects corruption or waste because budgets do not generally indicate how funds are related to service delivery targets. In addition, the budgets themselves may be deliberately shaped to facilitate corruption. For example, managers may budget for unnecessary workshops so that they can collect per diems or may prioritize spending on new office furniture instead of patient education programs. Traditional financial monitoring will not identify such abuses.

Weak record keeping makes it difficult to monitor financial performance. For example, studying 23 countries with hospital user fee systems, Barnum and Kutzin (1993) found that in only two countries did hospitals keep records which would allow fee collection information to be matched to service utilization (Barnum and Kutzin 1993). Virtually no hospitals kept track of total patients exempted from paying fees. A study in Kenya found that 78% of fees actually earned by one provincial hospital went uncollected. There was no record that patients had paid fees for the services they received, or, if they did pay, that the fees were received by the facility. Similarly, in government facilities in Guinea, it was impossible to determine collection rates because patients who cannot pay are not registered as having received services (Newbrander et al. 2000).

Another problem is that financial and service delivery systems are traditionally managed separately, with finances being the responsibility of financial managers or accounting staff, and service delivery the responsibility of clinicians and technical managers. One African nurse manager described her relationship with the accounts office quite simply: "We work the wards, they go to meetings." Such professional boundaries, combined with a lack of management training, make it hard to produce accurate, timely financial performance indicators and use them properly. The introduction of performance-based financing in some countries has potential to bring about improvements, but systems remain weak. In Lesotho, program-based budgeting has been in place for several years, yet actual expenditures are not recorded by program in the accounting system and managers cannot monitor program performance against the budget (Vian 2009).

To effectively monitor financial performance, we need information on how resources have been used to achieve results. By combining financial data with service statistics, performance indicators such as average revenue and cost per service can be produced and compared with targets or standards, or with equivalent performance indicators at other facilities. When transmitted to senior managers and oversight bodies in a timely fashion, the results can prompt discussion and action, as shown in the case study that follows.

The Case of South Africa

One country that has taken advantage of financial performance monitoring to promote greater accountability and transparency in the health sector is South Africa. Four years after the fall of apartheid, the South African health-care system had many governance problems, including a lack of citizen input and spending patterns that did not reflect the true health needs of the population. Budgeting was arbitrary, and record-keeping systems did not provide data to hold officials accountable for performance. At the district level, systems for planning, budgeting, accounting, and health information each existed, but they were weak and operated as silos, with little cross-communication. Service plans were created each year and then rarely referred to again. Budgets were compiled and then slashed, so that the resulting numbers did not correspond to the actual cost of services the districts were expected to provide. Reams of paper were used to complete required reporting; yet, there was no information to monitor performance in relation to the plans or budgets. As one district manager put it, "We had to change. We were frustrated with the health care system, and had no useful information to base management on. This had a radical impact on our ability to provide quality health services."

In 1997 the Department of Health embarked on a program to expand equitable access to primary health-care services. With support from a donor, the government wanted to build the capacity of district health teams to use resources more efficiently to address priority health needs.[1] In addition to public health programs such as immunization, reproductive health care, health promotion, and disease control, the district health teams manage hospital- and health center-based clinical care at hundreds of public facilities.

Action Plan

Accountability for health-care system performance demands that public officials use resources wisely to achieve objectives. To provide transparency on this process, one must look at expenditure in relation to what was produced. The district manager, information officer, and finance officer needed to work together to see the relationships between how resources are allocated and how they are used to produce services. The key to increasing accountability in district health management would be to link planned and actual services to the resources used to achieve them and to compare performance over time, with targets and across similar facilities. Because many of the staff in health districts were untrained in management, it was important to start with a simple system.

The project began by introducing a district health planning and reporting system as part of the rollout of the medium-term expenditure framework by the Department of Health. This centered around an annual review and analysis of health services and financial performance, including key indicators such as the number of services per day (in total and per nurse), cost per patient visit and bed day (total and supplies), cost of staff, drugs, and maintenance, and user fee revenue per patient discharge. These indicators were compared over 3 years, with targets and across similar facilities.

The plans and annual reports were sent to municipal government, other district teams, and the Provincial Department of Health, providing the opportunity for external, peer, and hierarchical review and enhanced accountability. Each facility and district was also required to monitor and report on its performance on a monthly basis and the reports were reviewed quarterly. Additional monitoring systems were introduced, covering related areas such as facility supervision. With project assistance, the National Department of Health implemented the district health planning and reporting systems nationwide and produced a written manual as a reference tool for district management teams (National Department of Health, Republic of South Africa 2003).

Results

The government compared financial and performance data at several levels in order to detect problems. The implementation took time and required a lot of training and technical assistance for planning and budgeting in each of the districts. Management teams eventually produced annual district reports with indicators that combined financial and utilization data, in most cases for the first time.

In "Tanbela District," staff calculated the cost of medicines per visit at each clinic and compared them as shown in Figure 12.1.[2]

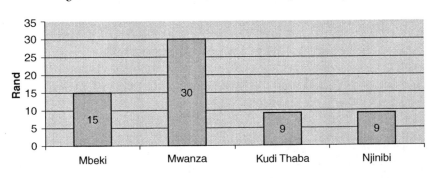

Figure 12.1 Tanbela district, medicine cost per visit by clinic

Figure 12.2 Batarana district, hospital expenditure per inpatient day

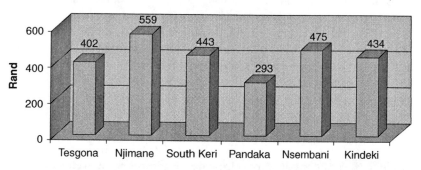

Staff found that medicine consumption was very high in Mwanza Clinic, over three times the medicine cost per visit in two other centers. The results were surprising and provoked much discussion. Although there could be a reasonable explanation for the high expenditure on drugs for Mwanza, such as a different mix of services, without this initial analysis, no one would have thought to ask questions. The information allowed managers to probe for potential abuse or diversion of resources, inefficiencies, or compelling reasons why expenditures should be legitimately different from the average. Comparison of total medicine expenditure per clinic would not have been as useful as the per-visit comparisons, since total expenditure does not take into account the different numbers of patient visits at individual clinics.

"Batarana District" applied similar financial performance monitoring techniques, comparing cost per unit among hospitals (see Figure 12.2).

District staff observed a higher-than-average expenditure in Njimane Hospital. The performance report provided the basis for animated discussions to probe the reasons for the high expenditure. Some of the questions which people raised included the following: What portion of Njimane Hospital's costs are "controllable," that is, what portion of costs can the management team actually influence through their own decisions? Did the hospital treat fewer patients than expected in that year, or did patients stay for fewer days than expected, thus leading to a higher cost per bed day? Were costs higher because hospital personnel wasted resources, or did they carry out more tests, which resulted in better quality of care? The graph alone does not answer these questions, but for the first time, it allowed supervisors to raise them, holding hospital managers accountable for explaining the operational decisions or contextual factors which led to the higher costs.

Managers were able to "drill down" to examine some types of expenditure in more detail. They were worried in particular about food costs, since a high cost per meal could indicate inflated prices charged by private catering services contracted by the hospital, or procurement of excess food so that some could be diverted. The managers discovered that the cost per patient meal was highest at Njimane Hospital and decided to focus their supervision in this area.

Comparing across facilities is helpful to identify anomalies in spending, but what if all the facilities were under-spending or over-spending? To identify this type of problem, one must compare expenditures to a norm or standard. This concern led the district of "Gauteng" to carry out a more detailed analysis of actual clinic expenditures compared to standard costs (Collins and Lewis 2003). The standard costs were developed by an expert panel of practitioners for each type of service and are based on estimates of the quantities of staff time, drugs, tests, and operating costs that were required to provide good-quality services. A simple calculation of the average cost per service showed that one of the clinics spent more than twice as much as the others. However, the standard cost analysis showed that the "over-spending" clinic needed more resources than the other clinic because it had a different service mix, which included greater quantities of higher-cost services. So part of the difference in expenditures could be explained by the service mix. Interestingly, both of the clinics were receiving much less funding than they actually needed to provide the services—even the clinic which appeared to be over-spending was, in fact, under-funded.

While South Africa has made great strides in implementing financial performance monitoring in the health sector, progress has been hampered by a lack of appropriate service statistics. For example, while data on total health centre visits were collected through the health information system, the data did not permit managers to drill down by type of visit. Health data systems designed to measure disease prevalence and cure rates may not have adequate data to measure a facility's productivity and efficiency. To address this problem, a "tick" register was introduced with columns showing the total number of each type of service delivered. By strengthening the systems used to report service statistics, managers are better able to "peel the onion" of unit cost data and identify root causes of performance problems, assuring full accountability of government agents in charge.

Conclusion

The need for management control systems and tools is increasing as more governments move toward decentralization and contracting out for health services. South Africa's efforts to improve performance and expenditure tracking at provincial and district levels have resulted in better management control, providing useful information with which to hold government agents accountable. The success in South Africa thus far shows that what you measure really does affect what people do. Instead of allowing financial personnel to be accountable for budgets while medical personnel are accountable for services, a system that brings together the locus of responsibility for costs and outputs, holding the service manager accountable, is essential in order to curb corruption.

Notes

1. EQUITY Project, 1997–2003, with funding from USAID.
2. Figures in this chapter use real data but with disguised district and clinic names.

References

Barnum, H., and J. Kutzin. 1993. *Public hospitals in developing countries: Resource use, cost, financing.* Baltimore, MD: The Johns Hopkins University Press.

Collins, D., and E. Lewis. May 2003. *A cost analysis of primary health care services.* Boston, MA: The EQUITY Project, Management Sciences for Health.

National Department of Health, Republic of South Africa. 2003. Guidelines for District Health Planning and Reporting. www.doh.gov.za/docs/factsheets/guidelines/dhp/index.html.

Newbrander, W., D. Collins, and L. Gilson. 2000. *Ensuring equal access to health services: User fee systems and the poor.* Boston, MA: Management Sciences for Health.

Vian, T. 2009. Good governance and performance based budgeting: Factors affecting reform progress in Lesotho hospitals. PhD dissertation, Boston University, Boston, MA.

Further Reading

Collins, D., Z. Jarrah, and P. Gupta. February 2009. *Cost and funding projections for the minimum package of activities of the Ministry of Health, Royal Government of Cambodia.* The BASICS Project (USAID). This report describes a recent example of using the standard costing approach.

Management Sciences for Health. 2009. The current version of the tool used to estimate standard costs is called CORE Plus. The tool and a manual can be found on the Financial Management page of the Health Manager's Toolkit at http://erc.msh.org/toolkit/.

Management Sciences for Health. *The Equity Project 1997–2003: Final report* (50 pp.). Boston, MA: Management Sciences for Health. Download by clicking on .pdf file link (2.5 MB) at www.msh.org/programs/southafrica_equity.html.

National Department of Health, Republic of South Africa. The website of the Department of Health contains many documents of interest, including *Financial management: An overview and field guide for district management teams* (April 2002). www.doh.gov.za/docs/reports/2002/finance/index.html.

Shah, A., and C. Shen. 2007. A primer on performance budgeting. In *Budgeting and budgetary institutions*, ed. A. Shaw, chap. 5, 137–178. Public Sector Governance and Accountability Series. Washington, DC: World Bank.

Soeters, R., and F. Griffiths. 2003. Improving government health services through contract management: A case from Cambodia. *Health Policy and Planning* 18, no. 1:74–83.

WHO has several sets of useful guidelines and documents relating to health resource planning and analysis available at www.who.int/management/resources/finances/en/index.html.

CHAPTER 13

Budget Transparency, Civil Society and Public Expenditure Tracking Surveys

William D. Savedoff and Ethan Joselow

Introduction

Governments play a significant role in providing or financing health-care services, yet too often the link between spending and outputs is weak. When governments spend substantial amounts on health care but services remain limited and of poor quality, these are signs of poor governance. The state may be spending on the wrong things or in the wrong places, it may be wasting resources through inefficient administration and management, or it may be losing money through corrupt practices. Whatever the reason, the result is ineffective programs, which limit the amount and quality of health-care services that are accessible to the public.

Ensuring that public funds are used well to increase access to health-care services and improve population health is not easy and is not something that can be done in a single reform. It involves not only a country's laws, regulations, and bureaucratic institutions but also its politics and mechanisms for public accountability. By collecting, publicizing, and using information about government spending, the public can constrain opportunities for corruption and pressure official institutions to fulfill their responsibilities.

While Chapter 12 explores the role of financial performance monitoring in improving the transparency and accountability of public spending, this chapter explores the role of public disclosure in the same endeavor. It presents a framework for understanding accountability that highlights the importance of information and transparency. It then discusses ways that countries have made public expenditures transparent, and ways that civil society can pressure governments to be more open. The chapter concludes with a discussion of Public Expenditure Tracking Surveys (PETS), an approach to identifying problems in public financial management when government cannot or will not collect and process public budget and expenditure information.

Public Spending, Transparency, and Accountability

In order to improve public spending, we need to understand the relationships between politicians and policymakers, providers of services, and citizens (see Figure 13.1). In private markets, health-care providers are directly accountable to the people who use, and pay for, their services. Not so with publicly provided or financed health care. Instead, providers in public systems are accountable to the government. If the government owns and operates its own health-care system, then providers are accountable to politicians and policymakers through a range of managerial and bureaucratic mechanisms. If the government pays for health services, the providers are still accountable to the government, but through contractual relationships. When citizens are not satisfied with the services they receive, they can voice their concerns to providers, but their main channel of accountability operates through politicians and government agencies. Citizens can complain to a local district health office, write to the Minister of Health, or pressure their legislators and other governmental representatives with petitions, letters to newspapers, and votes.

A large number of public reform efforts try to create direct accountability of public providers to citizens by offering channels for direct feedback, giving citizens vouchers to reward better-performing providers, or creating supervisory boards with citizen input. Other policies focus on making

Figure 13.1 A generalized framework for accountability

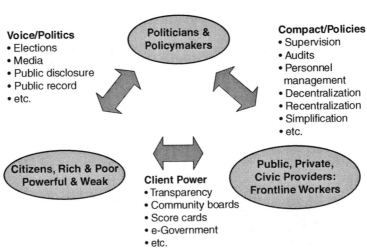

Source: Adapted from World Bank, *World Development Report, 2004.*

government finances transparent so that people can see how taxpayers' money is being used. Only when public budget and expenditure information is available for scrutiny can citizens effectively pressure their government to use money well.

Studies have shown a significant relationship between budget transparency and the quality of governance. For example, countries with better public information on budgets, as indicated by having freedom of information laws, also demonstrate better overall governance (Islam 2003). Public budget transparency is positively associated with higher national income (International Budget Partnership [IBP] 2008; see Figure 13.2), and countries with more transparent budgets generate more trust and confidence, allowing them to borrow from international bond markets at less cost than those who are less transparent (Glennerster and Shin 2008).

A first condition for citizens to be able to hold their government accountable is public availability of budget and expenditure information. Financial information can be very complex and most citizens lack the time or expertise to analyze it, so a second condition is that information must be available in a clear and useful format. Even with easy-to-use information, eliciting responses from governments requires some form of institutional representation through political parties, nongovernmental organizations

Figure 13.2 Open budget index and its relationship to GDP

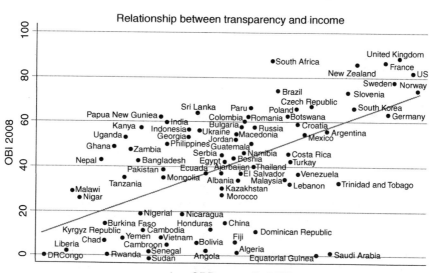

Source: IBP (2008).

(NGOs), or civil society organizations (CSOs). With public information that is clear and useable, civil society can begin to monitor budgets and expenditures and appropriately pressure the government to handle taxpayers' money responsibly.

The First Step: Access to Useable Information

In most democracies, citizens have some rights to information about how the government functions, though in many countries these rights are heavily circumscribed or the government fails to fulfill them. Increasingly, it is expected that government should grant civil society access to accurate and timely information on how budget decisions are made, as well as the outcomes of spending for beneficiaries. Yet, the IBP's 2008 Open Budget Survey found that of 85 countries surveyed, only 5 made extensive, detailed information available to the public and in the 23 lowest-performing countries, the public had no access to budget proposals before approval (IBP 2008).

There are many ways to improve access to information about government budgets and spending. In the simplest cases, willing governments need only publish existing information. Sometimes regulations need to be changed or laws passed, permitting this information to enter the public domain. But in many countries, basic legislation is required to establish the principle that the government information is public information, that is, that the burden should be on the government to prove why information should be withheld rather than on citizens to prove why it should be available.

One way that countries have started this process is to pass freedom of information laws. Mendel (2004)proposes nine legal principles that, if enacted and followed, provide a sound basis for giving the public access to the information it needs to hold government accountable for its use of public funds (see Box 13.1). The first of these is the principle of maximum disclosure, which establishes "a presumption that all information held by public bodies should be subject to disclosure and that this presumption may be overcome only where there is an overriding risk of harm to a legitimate public or private interest"(Mendel 2004, 30).

While the standards for public transparency are well known, relatively few countries actually meet them. Even in countries such as France, South Africa, and the United Kingdom, which have high transparency, budget and expenditure information needs to be processed and explained before it is useful. NGOs have been established in many places to fill this gap.

One example is the Public Services Accountability Monitor (PSAM—www.psam.org.za) that operates in the South African province of Eastern Cape. PSAM has expanded its anticorruption watchdog role to

---

Box 13.1   List of principles for freedom of information

1. *Maximum disclosure:* Freedom of information legislation should be guided by the principle of maximum disclosure.
2. *Obligation to publish:* Public bodies should be under an obligation to publish key information.
3. *Promotion of open government:* Public bodies must actively promote open government.
4. *Limited scope of exceptions:* Exceptions should be clearly and narrowly drawn and subject to strict "harm" and "public interest" test.
5. *Process to facilitate access:* Requests for information should be processed rapidly and fairly and an independent review of any refusal should be available.
6. *Costs:* Individuals should not be deterred from making requests for information by excessive costs.
7. *Open meetings:* Meetings of public bodies should be open to the public.
8. *Disclosure takes precedence:* Laws which are inconsistent with the principle of maximum disclosure should be amended or repealed.
9. *Protection for whistle-blowers:* Individuals who release information on wrongdoing must be protected.

Source: Mendel (2004).

---

include more comprehensive external monitoring of government agencies' strategic planning, financial management practices, and levels of accountability. PSAM analyzes the provincial budget, monitors how well actual spending follows it, and publishes this information in concise and standardized formats. To encourage the government to improve the quality of data provided, it has explicitly measured and publicized government transparency. For example, it created an evaluation template for the government's strategic planning process and regularly assesses and publicizes the government's performance.

Another example in which an NGO has pressured government to be more transparent can be found in Colorado (United States). The Colorado Fiscal Policy Institute (COFPI—www.cclponline.org) has outlined a series of principles for transparency and assesses the Colorado state government in its regular reports. One of the most powerful tools that COFPI employed was a "Budget Transparency Scorecard." The scorecard is a simple graphic representation of each of the principles and a measure of how well the government agency meets those principles (see Figure 13.3).

In sum, while legal changes such as the enactment of freedom of information laws can make budget information available to the public, such policy changes are often insufficient on their own. The general public

Figure 13.3 Scoring Colorado's state government on budget transparency

GRADE	SCORING SUMMARY	AREAS OF EVALUATION	SCORE	GRADE
√√√√	Colorado's budget substantially complies with recommended practices	I. Availability in (governor's) proposed budget of revenue, expenditure, and fund balance data—historical and projected	52/152 (34%)	√
√√√	Colorado's budget complies with recommended practices most of the time	II. Availability of revenue, expenditure, and fund balance projections as budget proceeds through the legislative process	20/29 (69%)	√√
√√	Colorado's budget complies with some of the recommended practices	III. Availability of information to put budget data in context	35/97 (36%)	√
√	Colorado's budget minimally or seldom complies with recommended practices	IV. Availability of supplemental tax and revenue information	2/34 (6%)	–
–	Colorado's budget generally does not comply with recommended practices	V. Budget process issues	9/38 (24%)	√

Source: Zelenski (2003).

cannot hold government to account if that information is obfuscated by jargon, difficult to access, or otherwise unclear. When governments fail to provide useable information, citizens and NGOs acting on their behalf can step into process and present the information in clear formats and pressure governments to be more open by publicizing transparency performance measures.

From Useable Information to Advocacy and Action: Examples in Mexico and India

The role of civil society in holding governments accountable involves more than just publishing clear, concise information on budgets and administrative processes. Interest groups must also organize members of the general public to exert pressure on authorities, all while retaining a trustworthy public profile. A collaborative relationship between organized NGOs, social movements, academics, and the media is a crucial component of a powerful, transformative movement for government accountability (Robinson 2006). There is also a need for capacity building among members of the public—equipping people with the tools necessary to be advocates for transparency.

Many organizations around the world are undertaking these tasks: monitoring government budgets and expenditures, publishing simple-to-understand reports, training people to use the information, and engaging in advocacy to hold government accountable. Two of these organizations are Fundar in Mexico and DISHA (Developing Initiatives for Social and Human Interaction—www.disha-india.org) in India.

Fundar—Mexico

Since 1999, a Mexican NGO called Fundar (www.fundar.org.mx) has effectively used requests under Mexico's freedom of information laws and electronic information available through the Federal Institute for Access of Public Information (IFAI) to monitor government budgets and spending. One of its projects investigated the use of public money in the fight against HIV/AIDS.

During the 2002 budget process in Mexico, the President of the Budget Committee of the Chamber of Deputies requested that the Ministry of Health divert M$30 million to eight NGOs to assist women and the minister complied. Many protested in Congress because the diversion was arbitrary and irregular. Alerted to the controversy, Fundar used freedom of information provisions to discover that the NGOs were linked to a pro-life group, Provida, that opposes government policies—such as safe sex—aimed at halting the HIV/AIDS epidemic. Fundar found that 90% of the funds were misused and some of the NGOs were "ghost" organizations. In response to Fundar's publications and advocacy, the government compelled Provida to return the funds and pay a large fine (M$13 million). It was also barred from receiving public funds for the next 15 years (de Renzio and Krafchik 2007).

Fundar also discovered that federal money dedicated to HIV/AIDS programs was being allocated into general funds and spent on line items such as building maintenance or financial services. Fundar used press conferences to leverage meetings with department heads and the internal comptroller, and two congressional committees. Fundar succeeded in increasing funding for HIV/AIDS prevention, while contributing to a change in administrative practices that were at the root of inefficiencies and lax oversight.

Developing Initiatives for Social and Human Interaction—India

Another NGO that effectively combines monitoring public spending and advocacy is DISHA. Since its founding in 1985, DISHA has worked to strengthen the economic and political position of Gujarat's poorest communities, found mostly among the tribal and lower-caste "dalit"

Box 13.2   Strategies for each phase of the public spending cycle

Even in the absence of freedom of information laws, DISHA has been able to pressure the Gujarat government to fulfill its commitments to the state's disadvantaged communities. It achieves this by using distinct strategies for each of four phases in the Gujarat spending cycle.

Budget formulation: Formulation of the Gujarat budget is not transparent and is decided in closed meetings. To increase attention to the needs of the poor, DISHA meets during this phase with legislators, develops press articles, and makes specific policy recommendations that they would like to see implemented.

Budget approval: The debate and approval of the budget plan is an opportunity for DISHA to write and publish commentaries on the governor's and the finance minister's statements, budget priorities, and budget trends. DISHA develops questions and talking points for legislators to respond to and question budget line items.

Budget execution: During budget execution, popular involvement is crucial. DISHA informs local leaders of the allocations for budget items in their jurisdiction and follows up with those leaders to ensure that the work took place according to the budget's allocations. In addition, DISHA trains local groups to monitor and report on expenses and it disseminates information about execution.

Evaluation and audit: Gujarat does not facilitate public access to information from the executive branch and external auditors regarding actual expenditures and the effectiveness of spending. So DISHA performs its own comparisons of budget descriptions with locally collected information on how the budget was implemented and disseminates this information to NGOs, legislators, and the media.

Source: Malajovich and Robinson (2006).

---

populations of the state. With a history of heavy involvement in areas of social activism such as land tenure rights, women's rights, and the unionization of laborers, DISHA found that bringing traditionally unempowered constituencies into budget discussions could have a substantial impact on their lives (Malajovich and Robinson 2006) (see Box 13.2).

One of DISHA's efforts is aimed at ensuring that government departments spend funds that have been allocated to social programs such as the Tribal Sub-Plan (TSP), which promotes the socioeconomic advancement of indigenous peoples. DISHA's strategy is to find out how much the state budget has allocated to specific projects and ask local government officials if the projects have been implemented. When it finds that projects are not being implemented, DISHA pressures the federal government to find out why and remedy the situation. Before DISHA got involved, the TSP budget was underspent by 20% (1993). By 1996, underspending was no longer a problem and many observers attributed this change to DISHA and its affiliates (de Renzio and Krafchik 2007). DISHA has trained NGOs and local governments in budget monitoring techniques and become a well-respected authority in state budget matters. By increasing public sector accountability, DISHA has shifted state budget priorities and spending in favor of the poor.

When All Else Fails: Track the Money

In many countries, holding government accountable for its use of public money is difficult because the government's own internal financial management is so inadequate. When the normal budget process does not generate or deliver the information, other approaches are needed. In some cases, citizens can be enlisted to report on whether funds are reaching their intended uses, an approach used by DISHA (see above). Another approach is to contract technical experts to do surveys and track public spending, using a PETS. This tool is useful where social service financial management and control is lacking.

The first PETS was conducted in Uganda in the mid-1990s, motivated by a puzzle: social spending was increasing but education and health services did not seem to improve. By conducting a representative survey of schools, the researchers found that, between 1991 and 1995, only 13% of the funds meant to provide education supplies in primary schools were actually reaching their intended uses (Ablo and Reinikka 1998). To date more than 24 PETS have been conducted with similar approaches and findings. For example, health districts with higher allocations in Chad allegedly provided fewer consultations. By tracking expenditures, however, one study showed that most of the federal money allocated to health facilities was being diverted, possibly stolen, and the gap between allocations and disbursements explained the low levels of productivity (Gauthier and Wane 2007).

Public expenditures can be tracked by comparing disbursements and receipts at any stage of the financial management process (see Figure 13.4) since every stage presents opportunities for diverting funds to legitimate or illegitimate uses (Savedoff 2008). For example, funds can disappear in transfers from federal to state governments, depicted as the difference between level 1 disbursements and level 2 inflows in Figure 13.4; they can disappear between local governments and health centers (e.g., between level 3 and facilities); or they can be diverted within a particular level (e.g., funds arriving at level 2 are stolen and never become an outflow).

Figure 13.4 Representation of potential leakage points

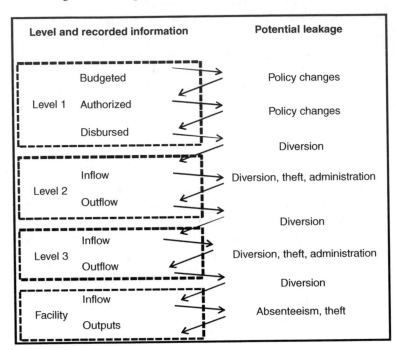

To get this information, expenditure tracking surveys generally collect a range of information, including the following[1]:

- Detailed descriptions of how funds are supposed to flow through the system, from the national treasury to frontline providers.

- Data from selected units at the national and subnational levels—including administrative data and interviews.

- Data from facilities—through administrative data or structured questionnaires and with purposive or representative samples.

- Information of how things "really work" from interviews with service providers, facility managers, officials at different government levels, and others outside government.

- Analyses of whether spending reaches facilities and is applied to its intended uses.

- Other findings regarding such things as delays in spending, problems in obtaining information, and equity.

- Recommendations regarding information systems, publicizing government budget data, increasing supervision, introducing new accounting instruments, and changing the institutional channels for financial flows, among others.

Expenditure tracking surveys have been conducted in more than 20 countries in the last decade. The most widely studied sector is education, followed by health. The health sector studies commonly find that federal money that is destined for wages is generally less vulnerable to diversion than are nonwage transfers, because wages are usually deposited directly in employees' bank accounts. By contrast, nonwage funds that flow through different levels of government are quite vulnerable to diversion. In many countries, funds seem to be diverted and misused at the local level—such were the findings in Mozambique, Senegal, and Rwanda—whereas in a few cases (Chad and Ghana), the most significant leakages were at the national level. Another general finding is that in-kind deliveries (e.g., drugs, medical supplies) are more susceptible to leakage than are financial transfers, partly because the monetary value of in-kind transfers is less transparent.

In Senegal, the central government pays local health workers directly but finances recurrent nonwage expenditures through a special fund, the Fonds de Dotation de la Décentralisation (FDD). By comparing records of funds disbursed from the FDD with records of funds received by local governments, one study was able to demonstrate serious leakages—due either to mismanagement or abuses. Medical regions in Dakar and Thiès received only 4% and 13%, respectively, of the money allocated to them under the FDD. Rwanda also found substantial loss of funds as money was transferred from one governmental level to the next. On average, only 76% of the funds disbursed by the central government were received by Regional Health Offices (RHOs). At the next stage, even more money seemed to disappear, with only 4–51% of RHO funds arriving at the country's District Health Offices (DHOs) (Fofack et al. 2003).

In Mozambique, an expenditure tracking study conducted in 2002 found that the volume of drugs distributed should have been sufficient to cover the requirements of public sector facilities. Nevertheless, more than half of all facilities reported that they lacked essential drugs at some time in the previous 6 months. These stock-outs lasted for 6–7 weeks on average, but in some cases were as long as 20 months. The study attributed the gap between drugs distributed and available to poorly understood rules and criteria for managing drug supplies. The study could not determine, however, whether the cause was mismanagement or theft (Lindelöw et al. 2004).

Knowing the problem is only part of its solution. In order to make a real, lasting impact, PETS and other surveys must be combined with policy recommendations that lead to a more productive set of incentives, better flows of information, and greater accountability for those in charge of public resources (Savedoff 2008). While technical studies such as PETS can uncover information for holding governments accountable, the information has to be disseminated and used by political actors if it is going to be a deterrent to those who would abuse public funds.

Conclusion

Finding out how much money governments allocate and spend is not easy, but it is key to holding public officials accountable for the effective use of taxpayers' money and to constraining opportunities for abuse. The first step is to establish the principle that information about the public sector belongs to the public and not to particular government officials. From there, it is necessary to transform public budget and expenditure information into easily understood and useable formats. CSOs have played pivotal roles, both in translating complex financial information into easily understood pamphlets and in using that information to uncover corruption and mismanagement. When the government itself cannot manage its finances, information can be collected through alternative means such as surveys and special audits to ascertain whether funds are reaching intended service delivery points. In these ways, societies around the world are moving toward greater openness and transparency in their budgets and citizens are gaining greater leverage to keep their governments honest.

Note

1. This list is taken from Savedoff (2008).

References

Ablo, E., and R. Reinikka. 1998. Do budgets really matter? - evidence from public spending on education and health in Uganda. Policy Research Working Paper Series 1926, World Bank, Washington, DC.

Ali, M.A. 2006. Lack of transparency and freedom of information in Pakistan: An analysis of state practice and realistic policy options for reform. Open Society Institute International Policy Fellowship Program paper. pdc.ceu.hu/archive/00003129/01/mukhtarAli_f3.pdf (accessed July 29, 2009).

de Renzio, P., and W. Krafchik. 2007. *Lessons from the field: The impact of civil society budget analysis and advocacy in six countries.* Washington, DC: International Budget Project. www.internationalbudget.org/ PractitionersGuide.pdf.

Dülger, C., and J.B. Justice. 2007. Fiscal transparency for citizen empowerment: The case of DISHA. Presentation to the annual conference of the Association for Budgeting and Financial Management of the American Society for Public Administration, Washington, DC, October 27, 2007.

Fofack, H., C. Obidegwu, and R. Ngong. March 2003. Public expenditure performance in Rwanda: Evidence from a public expenditure tracking study in the health and education sectors. Africa Region Working Paper Series 45, World Bank, Washington, DC.

Gauthier, B., and W. Wane. 2007. Leakage of public resources in the health sector: an empirical investigation of Chad. Policy Research Working Paper 4351, Development Research Group, World Bank, Washington, DC.

Glennerster, R., and Y. Shin. 2008. Does transparency pay? *IMF Staff Papers* 55, no. 1:93–209.

International Budget Partnership (IBP). 2008. Open budgets transform lives: The Open Budget Survey 2008. www.openbudgetindex. org/index.cfm?fa=fullReport (accessed July 25, 2009).

Islam, R. 2003. Do more transparent governments govern better? Policy Research Working Paper 3077, World Bank, Washington, DC.

Lindelöw, M., P. Ward, and N. Zorzie. 2004. Primary care in Mozambique: Service delivery in a complex hierarchy. Africa Region Human Development Working Paper Series, World Bank, Washington, DC.

Malajovich, L., and M. Robinson. 2006. Budget analysis and social activism: The case of DISHA in Gujarat, India. Case study. International Budget Project. www.internationalbudget.org/India-DISHA.pdf (accessed August 2, 2009).

Mendel, T. 2004. *Freedom of information: A comparative legal survey.* Paris: UNESCO.

Organization for Economic Cooperation and Development. 2001. Best practices for budget transparency. www.oecd.org/dataoecd/33/ 13/1905258.pdf (accessed July 29, 2009).

Public Services Accountability Monitor (PSAM). 2004. Submission to Medium Term Expenditure Committee Hearings, Eastern Cape Treasury—25/26 November 2004. An evaluation of proposed budget allocations and draft strategic plans for the Eastern Cape Departments of Health and Social Development for the 2005/06 Financial Year. Grahamstown, Eastern Cape, South Africa.

Ramkumar, V. 2008. *Our money, our responsibility: A citizen's guide to monitoring government expenditures*. Washington, DC: International Budget Project.

Robinson, M. 2006. Budget access and policy advocacy: The role of nongovernmental public action. Institute of Development Studies Working Paper 279, Institute of Development Studies, Brighton, UK.

Savedoff, W. 2008. *Public expenditure tracking surveys: Planning, implementation and uses*. Submitted to the World Bank June 10, 2008. Portland, ME: Social Insight.

World Bank. 2004. *World Development Report 2004: Making services work for poor people*. Washington, DC: World Bank.

Zelenski, J.M. October 2003. *The transparency of Colorado's budget process: Is it open, understandable, and accessible to Coloradans?* Denver, CO: Colorado Fiscal Policy Institute. www.cclponline.org/pubfiles/transparency.pdf (accessed September 23, 2009).

Glossary

absenteeism. When someone employed to work is not present or attending to work during agreed-upon working hours. An absence may be legitimate if it is in accordance with personnel policies (e.g., vacation, sick leave, or other approved leave) in which case it is an excused absence. Unexcused absences can be a sign of shirking, dual employment, or ghost workers.

accountability. An obligation or willingness to accept responsibility and to account for one's actions by furnishing a justifying analysis or explanation. Holding individuals or organizations accountable requires at least three things: identifying to whom they are accountable, specifying what they are accountable for, and establishing the consequences of fulfilling or not fulfilling their obligations.

arbitrage (parallel trade). When drugs or supplies are purchased from the public sector at low, often subsidized, prices and resold at higher prices in the private market.

bid-rigging. A process of manipulating public bidding for goods or service contracts in order to inflate prices and/or direct work to a particular supplier. Bid-rigging can involve manipulating documents, restricting advertising, changing procedures, and inappropriately influencing those who make decisions.

bribery. Bribery is the act of offering someone money, services, or other valuables, in order to influence the decision or action of a public agent. Bribes are also called kickbacks, baksheesh, payola, hush money, sweetener, protection money, boodle, and other terms.

bureaucratic corruption. Corrupt acts that involve embezzlement or extortion by people working in the middle and lower ranks of the public bureaucracy. In addition to its economic costs to citizens, such bureaucratic corruption undermines the credibility of public services, distorts public policy, and privileges citizens who are willing to pay bribes.

collusion. Agreement between two or more people to deceive or defraud others.

conflict of interest. Conflict of interest arises when an individual with a formal responsibility to serve the public participates in an activity that jeopardizes his or her professional judgment, objectivity, and independence. Often this activity (such as a private business venture) primarily serves personal interests and can potentially influence the objective exercise of the individual's official duties.

discretion. Autonomous authority to make decisions or exercise power.

embezzlement. Misappropriation of property or funds legally entrusted to someone in their formal position as an agent or guardian.

financial corruption. A general term involving fraud, embezzlement, falsification of financial statements, or other manipulation of financial records or theft of financial assets for personal gain.

fraud. Intentional deception or misrepresentation in order to obtain illegal or illegitimate benefits.

ghost workers. The term for individuals who are officially on the public payroll but who do no work for their pay.

graft. Misuse of an official position for personal gain through knowledge of public policies or influencing public policy in order to benefit personally.

grand corruption. Corrupt acts that involve major embezzlement or exchange of resources such as bribes for advantages among elites at the highest levels of government and private industry. It is considered serious both because it generally involves large-scale losses to society and because leaders who act this way establish corruption as an accepted or justified social norm.

kickback. A payment from a client or supplier to an official who has arranged for them to win a procurement or service contract.

nepotism. Nepotism is a form of favoritism in which an official exploits his or her power and authority to procure jobs or other favors for relatives.

patronage. The term "patronage" refers generally to the support or sponsorship of a patron (wealthy or influential guardian) and includes legitimate forms, such as when patrons support the arts. When referring to corrupt practices, however, patronage refers to people who secure appointments to government jobs, promotions, and contracts for work based on personal or political connections rather than merit or qualifications.

petty corruption. Like bureaucratic corruption, petty corruption involves embezzlement or extortion by people working in the middle and lower ranks of the public bureaucracy. The term is usually applied to those situations in which bureaucrats interact directly with clients, for example, demanding payments to provide a service or complete an official procedure. Although petty corruption usually involves much smaller sums than those involving grand corruption, it is often the aspect of corruption that is most visible to and directly penalizes citizens.

political corruption. The term political corruption is sometimes used synonymously with "grand" or high-level corruption and refers to the misuse of entrusted power by political leaders. It may also refer specifically to corruption within the political and electoral processes.

principal–agent theory. A field of economics involving analysis of situations in which an agent is contracted to do work on behalf of another (the principal). Many studies of corruption use this theory to examine the behavior of officials who are entrusted to act on behalf of the public but who can also betray this trust through corruption.

rent seeking. An activity undertaken by an individual to enrich himself or herself from controlling a scarce resource (e.g., land) without contributing anything of value. When a public official enriches herself by manipulating her discretion over government decisions (e.g., in granting licenses), it is a form of corruption.

systemic corruption. Corruption is said to be systemic when it is an integrated and essential aspect of the economic, social, and political system, rather than occasional and extraordinary. Systemic corruption characterizes situations in which the major institutions and processes of the state are routinely dominated and used by corrupt individuals and groups, and in which most people have no alternatives to dealing with corrupt officials.

transparency. Transparency is the quality of being clear, honest, and open. As a principle, transparency implies that civil servants, managers, and trustees have a duty to act visibly, predictably, and understandably. Sufficient information must be available so that other agencies and the general public can assess whether the relevant procedures are followed, consonant with the given mandate. Transparency is therefore considered an essential element of accountable governance, leading to improved resource allocation, enhanced efficiency, and better prospects for economic growth in general.

theft. Illegal taking of another person's property or public property.

Source: Authors and the U4 Anticorruption Resource Centre (www.u4.no).

Contributors

Taryn Vian, MS, PhD, is Assistant Professor of International Health at the Boston University School of Public Health and a recognized international expert on corruption in the health sector. She teaches a graduate course in Preventing Corruption in Health Programs and has facilitated professional training seminars on anticorruption in several countries. Vian assessed vulnerabilities to corruption in Albania and Azerbaijan and has done field research on the problem of informal payments for health services in Albania. Her recent work is on financial management reform to increase accountability in government health services in Lesotho. She writes widely on the topic of health sector corruption, and her articles have been published in *Health Policy & Planning*, *Social Science & Medicine*, and the *International Encyclopedia of Public Health*.

William D. Savedoff, PhD, is Senior Partner at Social Insight, an international consulting firm with expertise in economic and political analysis of public policy, and a Visiting Fellow at the Center for Global Development in Washington, DC. A former senior economist at the Inter-American Development Bank, Savedoff worked with coeditor Rafael Di Tella to produce *Diagnosis Corruption: Fraud in Latin America's Public Hospitals*, a book presenting seven case studies analyzing bribes, theft, absenteeism, and overcharging for supplies in hospitals. He recently conducted an assessment of vulnerabilities to corruption in the health sector in Ethiopia, and consults frequently for the World Bank, IDB, U4 Anticorruption Resource Centre, and other international organizations.

Harald Mathisen, MA, is a political scientist with a wide geographical and topical experience in the field of governance and anticorruption. As Senior Project Coordinator and now Acting Director of U4 Anticorruption Resource Centre in Bergen, Norway, for 6 years he has been engaged in developing and facilitating workshops on anticorruption and good governance, coordinating research projects, conducting analyses, and developing strategies related to anticorruption topics. He has published extensively and presents regularly at conferences and seminars on anticorruption strategies and the work of the international community in this field.

David H. Collins, FCA, MA, is Director of Finance and Accounting at the corporate level for Management Sciences for Health. He also does short-term consulting in health finance in many countries and was a long-term advisor on USAID-funded health sector reform projects in South Africa and Kenya.

Ethan Joselow, MPH, is a research associate at the Georgia State University's Andrew Young School of Policy Studies. He has several years' experience in US health services research and health policy and has conducted primary research on health sector corruption in India.

Ottar Mæstad, PhD, is senior researcher and economist at Chr. Michelsen Institute (CMI) in Norway and head of CMI's research program on Global Health and Development. He has examined issues of governance, health and economic development, and the economics and ethics of priority setting in health and has led many research projects for clients including OECD, World Bank, and NORAD.

Kelly Miller is an MPH candidate in international health at Boston University School of Public Health. She has studied health disparities in Latin America and, upon completing her MPH, will serve as a public health volunteer for the United States Peace Corps in Guinea.

Stephen N. Musau, BCom, FCA, is a Kenyan chartered accountant working in Washington, DC, with Abt Associates Inc., where he is Health Financing Advisor for the Health Systems 2020 Project. He has more than 20 years of experience in consulting with governments on health systems strengthening, including health financing, human resources for health, and policy development. He has also worked as a financial auditor and tax advisor in Kenya and the United Kingdom.

Aziza Mwisongo, MD, PhD, is a Tanzanian health system researcher based at the National Institute of Medical Research in Dar es Salaam. Her research focuses on health sector reforms, human resources for health, equity, health systems performance, and policy analysis.

Nancy Scott, MPH and DrPH candidate, is a research associate with the Center for Global Health and Development at Boston University School of

Public Health. She has extensive experience in managing research projects in field sites in the developing world.

Katherine Semrau, MPH, PhD, has worked in Africa for 4 years on a variety of maternal and child health projects. She focuses mainly on infectious disease epidemiology, especially HIV/AIDS, and research on improving child survival in low-resource settings.

Brenda Waning, MPH, RPh, serves as Director of Pharmaceutical Policy at Boston University School of Medicine. She has more than 10 years of experience in teaching, research, and consulting in the area of global pharmaceutical policy and access to medicines, with regional expertise in Central Asia. Her current research is focused on monitoring, predicting, and measuring impacts of various global policies and strategies on markets for antiretroviral and antimalarial medicines.

Index

Also from Kumarian Press...

Anticorruption and Governance:

The World Bank and the Gods of Lending
Steve Berkman

Where Corruption Lives
Edited by Gerald. E. Caiden, O.P. Dwivedi and Joseph G. Jabbra

Fighting Corruption in Developing Countries: Strategies and Analysis
Edited by Bertram Spector

Building Democratic Institutions: Governance Reform in Developing Countries
G. Shabbir Cheema

New and Forthcoming:

Rethinking Corporate Social Engagement: Lessons from Latin America
Lester M. Salamon

Dispossessed People: Establishing Legitimacy and Rights for Global Migrants
Christine Ho and James Loucky

Inside the Everyday Lives of Development Workers: Values, Motives and Aspirations
Heather Hindman and Anne-Meike Fechter

Civil Society Under Strain: Counter-terrorism, Civil Society and Aid Post-9/11
Edited by Jude Howell and Jeremy Lind

Visit Kumarian Press at **www.kpbooks.com** or
call **toll-free 800.232.0223** for a complete catalog

Kumarian Press, located in Sterling, Virginia, is a forward-looking, scholarly press that promotes active international engagement and an awareness of global connectedness.